A Woman's Heart

A Woman's Heart

Sex Matters!
Understanding the Number One killer of Women

A. Emrani, M.D.

iUniverse, Inc.
New York Lincoln Shanghai

A Woman's Heart
Sex Matters

iUniverse, Inc.

For information address:
iUniverse, Inc.
2021 Pine Lake Road, Suite 100
Lincoln, NE 68512
www.iuniverse.com

ISBN: 0-595-29743-9

Printed in the United States of America

Dedicated to my grandmothers, Tuba and Morvarid; my mother, Manijeh; my wife, Nooshin; and my daughter, Ariel.
These women have influenced my life deeply each generation.

CONTENTS

What Are You Doing With All Those Hearts?

One of the fondest memories of childhood is my mother chasing me across the yard. She wanted her chicken hearts back. I was quick-legged, nimble little sprite of a boy. I dodged and wove between the sheets on the clothesline, under the swings, down the slide. I had a precious possession to protect. To my mother, they were just chicken parts. To me, they were an initiation into the mysteries of the physical body.

I looked forward to the twice-monthly visits to the market, when she would buy a dozen chickens for her delightful cooking. So fascinated was I with the physical body that I would sneak in, steal the innards, and perform surgery on them in an attempt to understand how the pieces worked together.

A precocious child, surgery was my favorite pastime. Even at eleven, I knew I wanted to become a doctor. By the end of junior high school I was sure I wanted to learn how to fix the hearts of children. Eventually, this dream led to months of excruciating pediatric rotations at the University of California San Diego's School of Medicine.

This rotation was one of the most difficult experiences of my life. Children show such bravery and stoicism in the face of pain and illness, even when there seems to be little hope. They have unwavering faith in their parents and care-givers to heal them. Sometimes medicine has the answers, sometimes it doesn't. In any case, the process was always painful.

Haunted by the suffering I witnessed daily, I spent many nights in tearful reconciliation. I just didn't have the special faith and strength required to take care of sick children. I have always been a spiritual person, and I believe in a gracious God as a higher source of love. However, I also believe that the Achilles heel of any religious faith is the suffering of innocent children. I struggled for an answer. If I didn't follow the path of caring for children, what would I do?

Through a small miracle, I was scheduled for a short break in my rotations. I took the opportunity to get away from school and medicine and think about my future specialty. I spent many hours in discussion with my parents. One night, after a particularly in-depth conversation with my mother, I found the answer.

My mother was aging. Her hair was graying, and the small smile lines around her eyes had become what my grandfather called "character lines." It took her an extra push to get out of a chair, and she would get short of breath if she were too active. At one time, a fast little boy had been no match for her, but now it took extra effort to climb a flight of stairs. I realized her heart was likely a causative factor in these symptoms, and for a moment I felt as helpless as I had staring into the eyes of a dying child for the first time. In spite of this, my mother's graceful demeanor and love for her children persevered. The true nature of her heart could not be diminished.

I couldn't bear to work with suffering children because of their complete vulnerability, so I turned to working with women. They are the source of life. They carry children for the duration of pregnancy, experience the miracle of birth, and nurture our future generations. In medical school, women had been reduced to ovaries, a uterus, and their various disease states, but I knew a woman's heart was a much more complex organ.

I wanted to remain in the field of cardiology, but this time as a specialist in women; however, one thing troubled me. It was no secret that cardiology research was conducted on men, with the assumption that the only differences women presented were with respect to size. As a specialist in female hearts, could I blindly assume the pathology, microbiology, anatomy, and physiology of the heart applied equally to both sexes?

Some professors said, "What difference does it make? Are you trying to take us back in time and make us unequal?" Others, more interested and more honest, would say, "I don't know! But we only have one model" (that being the medical model based on men). Still fewer professors, encouraged by my curiosity, told me, "We need more research in that area, but the time hasn't come yet." I would find the answers to these questions in a couple of unexpected places.

Roberta, a warm, honest woman, was a hard-working mother of three. I first met her when I was assigned to her in one of the intensive-care rotations in my last year of medical school. Thanks to Roberta, I learned my first valuable lesson about women and the heart.

It was June when I first found her helpless in the ICU. Attached to several lines, drips, monitors, and life-support systems, she had been experiencing palpitations, dizziness, and fatigue since February. Her family and finances had gone through some major downturns in January, so her doctors, attributing her symptoms to the obvious, had diagnosed her with "stress" and "anxiety attacks."

By May, Roberta could not make it to the second story of her home without having to sit down and catch her breath. In June, when she was presented to the emergency room, she was unconscious, her lungs full of water, in such dire health that a respirator was necessary. Roberta, no longer able to breathe on her own, was on her way to requiring a heart transplant.

Far more serious than "stress," Roberta had developed cardiomyopathy, a condition of weakened muscle that causes the heart's pump to fail. Under this condition, the heart is unable to keep up with the demands of the body. In some, if discovered early enough, this condition can be medically treated. If found too late, however, the prognosis is grim, with complications usually leading to fatality. Not everyone with cardiomyopathy will be as fortunate as Roberta, nor will they necessarily be a candidate for a heart transplant.

During my residency, I also met Martha who had been complaining of palpitations for more than a decade. In part because she was verbose and determined, her physicians diagnosed her with anxiety disorder. The second time she lost consciousness, breaking a hip, her doctor finally considered a heart evaluation.

Her echocardiogram (the ultrasound of her heart), however, indicated a very different diagnosis. It showed a large tumor, the size of an apple, inside the upper chamber of her heart. Fortunately, via relatively simple surgery, this benign tumor was removed, and Martha was forever freed of her anxiety.

Since then, I have seen countless women with heart disease be ignored by professionals. Scientific studies have even shown us that while most women are concerned with breast cancer, far more die of heart disease.

I have made it my mission in my career, which is also my life's vocation, to work with women on the level they deserve. Science is just now learning how complicated and involved a woman's heart is. We are also learning that women's hearts are NOT like men's. Their physiologies and chemistries are entirely different, as are their risk factors, symptoms of disease, and necessary treatments.

Since childhood, I have had a deep appreciation for human life and a profound respect for women, feelings fostered by a loving mother and positive experiences with the women in my life. I learned from them, and from the many courageous women I see as patients, that women's hearts are closer to God and that their souls are more in tune with life.

Since choosing my own professional path, I have been honored to care for many brave women. I have been blessed with the ability to show them a better way of caring for themselves and their hearts. This book is an expression of love for my mother, who prepared me to embark upon this path, for my wife, who accompanies me, and for my daughter, who is the scalpel that pares away the unnecessary trimmings by her sheer innocence and trust. I wrote this book for you too, because at one time you will have been all these things to someone, somewhere. Those individuals love you and need you. Your paths will be varied, but your hearts must be strong for them and for yourself. Thank you for trusting me to show you the way.

CHAPTER 1

Myth versus Medicine

I can fix a broken heart, but only if I have all the essential pieces. I have the training to restart a heart after it has stopped and the required skills to surgically mend it when it is dying. I can repair damage caused by age and abuse. I can even help surgically transplant a totally new heart, fresh and young, to replace one that is worn past all functioning. However, this scientific knowledge means nothing if I don't have the right pieces with which to work.

As poetry often reminds us, a woman's heart is a complicated matter. Poets, musicians, and artists the world over have known for centuries what science is only just beginning to discover: there is much more to a woman's heart than muscle, tissue, and blood.

A woman's heart is the pulse of a family and the source of love. It is warmth, compassion, and nurturing. It is the core of physical passion and the center of a mother's instinct. A woman's heart demands special observation and careful consideration.

Up until recently, heart research had been performed exclusively on men. It was believed that pregnancy and fluctuating hormone levels would decrease the efficacy of the research, so women were automatically excluded from such studies. Also, heart-related drugs could not be tested on women of childbearing age lest they harm a developing fetus, a precaution that had roots in the thalidomide tragedy of the 1960s. So when a new discovery was made, it was assumed that women would respond in the same way as men, and they were treated accordingly. We now know this is not the case.

Although the feminist movement has made wonderful strides in empowering women in social arenas it inadvertently equated women with men in a physiological and biochemical sense. Women are not just men with "wo" in front of their gender name. Special attention must be given to their medical care, from presentation to treatment. Targeted funding is required for women's research, an initiative that starts with the understanding and appreciation of what sets men and women apart.

I have written this book to educate and inform women. It is a journey past the hard facts and cold data and into a deeper understanding of what the female heart symbolizes and how it is impacted by such factors as emotion, stress, hormones, age, and lifestyle. Your heart is uniquely female, as are the demands it experiences and the burdens it carries.

To illustrate this point, take a moment right now to place your hand over your chest. Do you feel the pulse? If you listen carefully, can you hear the beat?

When I take a patient's wrist and place my finger on her pulse point, I communicate with her on a deeper level. I know immediately if she is calm or anxious. My own slow pulse resonates with hers and she becomes relaxed. The gentle whooshing of her heart (the first sound babies hear in the womb) provides a sense of soothing.

Consider all of the idioms we sprinkle into our everyday conversations that incorporate this small mass of muscle: "learn by heart," "do one's heart good," "from the bottom of one's heart," "have one's heart in one's mouth," "have one's heart in the right place," "heart and soul," "heart of hearts," "lose heart," "wear one's heart on one's sleeve," "with all one's heart."

With such powerful images to draw from, it is no wonder we have neglected to understand the darker side. We don't want to admit a heart can be torn asunder by stress, anxiety, anger, and age. We desire that our mother's heart will last forever and that she will walk in front of us throughout our lives. We want her heartbeat to remain strong and steady, a beacon by which we find our way.

Admitting the heart's physical vulnerability is tantamount to facing our own mortality and the inevitable consequences of disease and aging. If we accept that something as awesome in power as a woman's heart can break, we must face the reality that so too can many things. We must admit our total dependence on a piece of muscle that weighs less than a pound and is no bigger than a fist.

I wrote this book to talk about all the ways we have to fix a broken heart, but I also hope to empower you to care for yourself on a deeper level. I want women to understand what has always been true and what science is just now getting around to explaining: women are wholly different from men, and their hearts, in particular, need specific care.

I am honored that you have chosen this book to guide you through the complicated world of medicine, cardiology specifically. I am pleased that you value yourself enough to take the initiative and learn as much as you can about your own health and how best to protect it.

This book is not a "prescription" on how to eat, exercise, and live. I don't purport to understand the complexities of your specific situation. I have simply consolidated the latest research and filtered it through my own medical education and experience in order to edify your scientific knowledge and provide you with a look inside the mysteries of the human body.

More importantly, I assert my personal belief that women are unique and should be cared for as such. From the beginning of time, women have been the life-givers and sustainers. Women's hearts carry a heavy burden.

Did you know that women are at greater risk for angina—chest pain and tightness—because the diameter of their blood vessels is typically smaller? We'll find out why and what you can do to help yourself.

We'll discuss the common heart problems, risk factors, and presentation of disease in women, along with the cutting-edge research in the field of cardiology. You will learn things your doctor probably doesn't know.

We take special care to discuss the emerging science with respect to Syndrome X and the role of inflammation in heart disease. We will deal with the complicated, confusing, and often misunderstood new research for hormone-replacement therapy in post-menopausal woman. These chapters alone will change everything you know about heart health and reinforce the gravity of the decisions you face when dealing with hormone-replacement therapy. Ample literature will show you that what you eat and how you exercise matter.

Finally, we will work through treatments and lifestyle changes that will keep your heart healthy. Women respond to testing as well as therapy differently than men. These differences need to be managed carefully and aggressively or they can have life-threatening implications.

I cannot remove the weight of your daily life; to do so would be to diminish your unequaled place in the world. I do, however, believe I can offer you valuable, enriching stories that are representative of women's lives today. It is my hope that these stories will connect with you. Along the way, you will become an informed healthcare consumer and an advocate for your own medical care.

Thank you for joining me on this journey. The world needs every woman's heart. It needs your heart.

CHAPTER 2

Sex Matters: The New Revolution

I want to start this chapter with a passage I first read in Robert Bly's book *Rag and Bone Shop of the Heart*. It was supposedly spoken by an Ethiopian woman to an anthropologist in an attempt to explain how men and women are different.

How can a man know what a woman's life is? A woman's life is quite different from a man's. God has ordered it so. A man is the same from the time of his withering. He is the same before he has sought out a woman for the first time, and afterwards. But the day when a woman enjoys her first love cuts her in two. She becomes another woman on that day. The man is the same after his first love as he was before. The woman is from the day of her first love another that continues all through life. The man spends a night by a woman and goes away. His life and body are always the same. The woman conceives. As a mother she is another person than the woman without child. She carries the fruit of the night for nine months in her body. Something grows. Something grows into her life that never again departs from it. She is a mother. She is and remains a mother even though her child dies. For at one time she carried the child under her heart. And it does not go out of her heart ever again. Not even when it is dead. All this, the man does not know; he knows nothing. He does not know the difference before love and after love, before motherhood and after motherhood. He can know nothing. Only a woman can know that and speak of that. That is why we won't be told what to do by our husbands. A woman can only do one thing. She can respect herself. She can keep herself decent. She must always be as her nature is. She must always be maiden and always be mother. Before every love she is a maiden, and after every love she is a mother. In this you can see if she is a good woman or not.

This passage speaks so richly and with such great symbolism that it says everything in a few pages that I will take an entire book to explain. On the surface, this woman's statements would appear to fly in the face of the modern women's liberation movement, but on the other it elevates women and sets them apart as being strong, mysterious, and powerful. A woman's health is intricately intertwined with every aspect of her emotional and spiritual well-being. This makes my job as a cardiologist fascinating, challenging, and occasionally frustrating. Science simply does not yet have all the answers we need when it comes to treating a woman's heart.

However, that is all about to change. The search for "equality" has netted women little in terms of medical research, but women's unique physiologic attributes are now becoming the "hot commodity" in the scientific community. We will be seeing many discoveries and breakthroughs in women's health in the coming years.

We Don't Test Women!

A study published in *Women's Health Issues* (Longo 1997) found that, interestingly enough, women are the major consumers of health care, the major consumers of prescription drugs, and the primary decision-makers about health care for their families. Even so, it wasn't until 1993 that the National Institute of Health's (NIH) Revitalization Act was put into place.

This act ensured that women and men were given equal time, participation, and consideration in medical research. Prior to that, there were two major biases present. 1) the male bias and 2) the male norm, which is the tendency to use men as the standard even in studies of diseases that affect both sexes.

> **Women's Health-Care Statistics**
> Leading Cause of Death (overall): Heart Disease—365,953 (2000)
> Number of Annual Office Visits to Physicians (all ages): 488 million (2000)
> Number of Annual Hospital Outpatient Department Visits: 50 million (2000)
> Number of Annual Emergency Department Visits: 57 million (2000)
> Number of Hospital Discharges (Inpatients): 19.2 million (2000)

With these two biases firmly entrenched, women simply were not being given equal time in the research world. They were looked upon as "small men." Women simply received smaller doses of drugs as adjusted for body size. Even with the advent of this act, sex and gender bias in heart-disease research and care is still among the most debated women's health issues.

Are We Really That Different?

Well, this can be a loaded question with controversial answers, so let's stick to what science has proven. Here are a few points to think about. Generally speaking—

♥ Some autoimmune diseases are much more prevalent in the female population, such as: Hashimoto thyroiditis, chronic active hepatitis, Graves' hyperthyroidism, systemic lupus erythematosus, scleroderma, rheumatoid arthritis, and multiple sclerosis (though rheumatoid arthritis and multiple sclerosis go into remission during pregnancy)

♥ Women have smaller lungs, even when adjusted for body size. Therefore, when women develop pulmonary disease such as asthma, lung cancer, or even sleep apnea, they have much more severe symptoms. Women smokers are also three times more likely to develop lung cancer than male smokers of the same age

♥ Over 44 million Americans have osteoporosis (bone density loss) and about 68% of them are women

♥ It takes longer for food to pass through a woman's digestive system than it does a man's

♥ Women have a higher incidence of gallstones

♥ Women suffer from irritable bowel syndrome about six times more often than men

♥ Women have a lower pain threshold but tolerate the pain better

Okay, But What about the Heart?

♥ Women are pharmacologically more sensitive to heart rhythm disturbances and more likely to develop torsades de pointes, a potentially deadly heart dysrhythmia

♥ Compared with men, women with cardiovascular disease report higher percentages of chronic pain, greater activity limitations, and more disability related to their disease (Heart and Stroke Foundation of Canada 1999)

♥ Women are two times more likely to die from a heart attack than men (Beery 1995, Shaffer and Corish 1998)

♥ Women were referred later and less often for CABG surgery (Beery 1995). When women were referred, they were older, sicker, more likely to have hypertension, diabetes, and hypothyroidism, and they have had higher mortality rates (Beery 1995; Shaffer and Corish 1998)

♥ Women have smaller hearts and smaller coronary arteries regardless of body size
♥ Women's heart rate generally responds faster to the same level of exercise
♥ A woman's blood has lower hemoglobin content

Signs and Symptoms of Heart Disease
- Shoulder or neck pain
- Nausea
- Fatigue
- Shortness of breath
- Spitting or coughing up blood
- Persistent cough
- Loss of consciousness
- Palpitations
- Swelling
- Bluish tinge to skin, particularly around the mouth

These are just a few of the known differences. More importantly, diagnosing heart disease in women can be a very tricky task. Because of this, women are more likely to be misdiagnosed and more likely to die from their first heart attack. In women, chest pain often presents as shoulder or neck pain, nausea, fatigue, or dyspnea, and lingering chest pain is found more frequently in younger, premenopausal women, with pain centered in neck or left arm rather than the typical substernal squeezing pain reported by men. Even if a woman does report the classic substernal-pressure symptom, it is less predictive of a heart attack than it would be in a man. When a woman develops heart disease, she—

♥ Typically presents at a later age
♥ Experiences more long-term disability
♥ Has a higher rate of additional disease processes
♥ Is less likely to undergo angioplasty or bypass surgery
♥ Is less likely to receive cardiac rehabilitation
♥ Is less likely to receive therapy with aspirin, beta-blockers, or ACE inhibitors

What about Testing?

If all of this weren't enough to make life very difficult for a cardiologist, testing women for cardiac disease adds another layer of complexity. It would be nice to think that in this age of technology we can immediately identify cardiac disease and/or heart attack in women. The matter is not that simple.

The exercise stress test is used with great success in diagnosed men but does not work as well for women. This test is performed by having a patient walk on a treadmill at predetermined levels of exertion and lengths of time. The patient is connected to an EKG monitor, which records the heart's activity. This test is noninvasive, relatively inexpensive, and until recently has been thought to work well for everyone. However, studies have shown that misleading test results occurred in about 35% of the women tested. There are many theories as to why this is the case, but none has yet bee proven. Some believe that the test is thrown off by the phases of the menstrual cycle, oral contraceptive use, and fluctuating hormone levels.

Pharmacologic stress tests are similar in concept but different in execution. In this case, the heart is forced to exert itself by drugs that are introduced to the system. For yet unknown reasons, these tests seem to be more predictive for women. In either case, the accuracy of the results is greatly improved if combined with echocardiography (an ultrasound of the heart).

Angiography is the process of introducing dye by way of a cardiac catheter. This allows the physician to identify blocked vessels by x-ray. This test works very well for men and women alike. However, as we read earlier, women are less likely to be referred for this test.

What Is the Medical Community Doing about These Differences?

To be honest, not enough, though changes are on the horizon. Emergency-room doctors miss diagnosing about 2% of patients having a heart attack or experiencing unstable angina because they do not have the "typical" symptoms. These people are frequently sent home and are twice as likely to die from their heart problems. Most of these patients are women under the age of fifty-five or minorities, who report shortness of breath as the concerning symptoms, rather than chest pain. Along with this, black women are much less likely than men or white women to receive life-saving therapies for heart attacks. They are also less likely to be referred for cardiac catheterization.

Clearly, the medical community has some room for improvement in these areas. The studies uncovering the misdiagnoses and misinterpretations are an excellent first step. We need to understand the problem before we can find a solution.

Women Are Under-treated

A study published in 2003 demonstrated that physicians often do not prescribe aspirin, beta-blockers, and cholesterol-lowering drugs to women after a heart attack. Some of the specific findings:

- Despite the high risk among the study participants, the use of medications for the prevention of a second heart attack was inadequate. Aspirin, beta-blockers, and cholesterol-lowering drugs are well-known tools to diminish the risk of a second heart attack. These drugs were substantially underused.
- Most of the women in the study were taking aspirin when the study began. However, only half were treated with beta-blockers, and only half who qualified for cholesterol-lowering drugs were using them.
- The women who had the greatest risk for heart disease were the least likely to be treated. (Vittinghoff 2003)

Why This Book?

I hope it has become clear from reading this chapter why it is vitally important to understand the differences between men and women, particularly with respect to the heart. Women need to be informed and educated so that they can adequately advocate for their own health care. You need to be clear on the implications your current actions may be having on your future heart health. Even if you are fortunate enough to have a health-care team that is up to date on the latest information in gender-based medicine, you still need to have an understanding for yourself. The decisions you make about activity and diet create ripples that will extend through many, many years of your life. Along with this, you are the front-line for diagnosing any looming problems. If you do not know what to look for with respect to heart-disease symptoms, you will not be able to effectively communicate impending difficulties to your physician. If you do not take seriously a symptom that may be signaling a heart attack, you are not likely to seek help in time.

I am not raising these issues in an attempt to divide men and women. I am not even seeking equality. I am only attempting to point out differences in order that women might take control of their own health issues and understand them for what they are. My main concern is that women feel educated and empowered enough that, when faced with a doctor that is not taking their symptoms seriously, they have the ability to hold firm and request the appropriate test or question an inappropriate medication. These decisions are not just important, they are vital. They spell life and death. You must take them seriously before you can expect anyone else to do so.

CHAPTER 3

The Perilous Heart: Risk Factors for Heart Disease

Sarah's Story

The alarm clock takes me out of a delicious dream. I am luxuriating in a bubble-filled bathtub with soft music playing, and, most importantly, I am ensconced behind a locked door. In real life, any mother knows what that means. It is the short time before the children start fighting and the door becomes the object that bears their frustration. "Mom, Johnny is hitting me!" "Mom, Stephanie won't give me back my space ranger toy!" But since this is a dream, I am able to fend off reality and enjoy the soothing feeling of the soft water and warm room, until the alarm rings. There is simply no way to tune out the annoying buzzer, especially after years of behavioral conditioning—alarm sounds, Sarah gets up, Sarah goes to work. There is no time to wake up slowly. It is time for the feet to hit the floor and greet the chilly morning, time to start the day and all the tasks that will become part of it.

The kids are sleeping soundly, and it takes several threats before they even open their eyes. There is breakfast to be made, lunches to be packed, school buses to be met, work clothes to be ironed—and all before heading into rush-hour traffic. The day has barely started and I'm already tired.

I do my best to negotiate traffic and listen to the news. I catch the guy in the car next to me giving me a dirty look. Seems he has a problem with my attempt to put on my lipstick and drive at the same time. I'm not sure what the issue is. We're in gridlock and moving nowhere, which brings me to the problem of my 8:00 meeting. No way I'm going to make it on time, but Josh let the cell phone go swimming in the toilet last night, and I have no way to call the office to let them know I'm on the way. I've had a very successful year, but my boss' patience is famously thin. It's a bit like treading on the last of the spring ice.

I really need to make this meeting on time. This is a huge client for us. Their business could represent a lot of money to the company and to my commission, which will help with the ever-mounting credit card bills. On top of it all, I need to remember to make an appointment with the dentist. I have a terrible toothache— most certainly a cavity—and it hurts enough that my stomach feels a bit nause- ated. No way I'm going to mess up this presentation because of a pain in my tooth, though. The show must go on. Finally the office is in sight, two minutes to spare, and I've already sweated through my shirt. Better remember to wear my jacket.

Does Sarah sound familiar? Can you recognize a bit of yourself in the tone of her life and speed with which events fly by? Maybe you work from home as a full-time mother and wife. Maybe you work two or even three jobs. Maybe you're retired and filling your days with one activity after another. Whatever the case, I think all women can relate to the pressure Sarah is feeling. The chaos of juggling so many things can be absolutely overwhelming. Women, in spite of themselves, are the caretakers and worriers, and their stress is compounded by the modern demands of work, family, and social life. Women have always felt these pressures. Even in most tribal environments, women bore tremen- dous responsibilities in terms of caring for children, gathering and preparing food, and protecting and raising livestock—and they did it all under very diffi- cult circumstances. Mere survival was the major challenge of each day.

In the industrial world, we don't struggle with physical survival on the same level, but our bodies haven't caught up to that fact yet. They still operate on the "fight-or-flight" instincts of our ancestors. Take Sarah as an example. If she were a primitive woman, her ears would be listening for the tiniest of sounds even as she slept. Any threat from a warring tribe or animal looking for a mid- night snack would slam her into wakefulness. Her hypothalamus would respond with a rush of adrenaline from the adrenal glands, and she would find herself able to run faster or fight stronger than she normally would. In the modern world, the alarm clock alone can stimulate this response, as it jars our senses and stimulates those instincts.

As Sarah goes about preparing for her day, she is assailed with any number of worries, or "stressors." For example, the thought of being reprimanded by her boss elevates her blood pressure and causes her heart to beat faster than normal. As she struggles through a sea of traffic, she suffers the same frustra- tion of salmon swimming upstream, trying valiantly to reach their spawning ground in order to propagate their species. The future survival of their species depends on their efforts, as does, in Sarah's mind, the future of her family and their well-being on her success at work, as well as her ability to juggle the myriad activities that come her way every day.

Keep Sarah in mind as you read through the more "technical" information of the next few chapters. Try to imagine her heart and circulatory system as you read about the science behind heart disease in women. Imagine how Sarah's lifestyle might contribute to her overall health (or lack thereof). We will be following her story, and the stories of other women, as we travel through these pages. In the end, I hope you will find inspiration and education, companionship and comfort. On the surface, there may be few similarities, but underneath you may find you are not so different. Learn from these women in order to help yourself, and in the end you will help others as well.

Taking Risks

There are worthy risks and then there are stupid mistakes. I hate to start off a discussion so bluntly, but the fact is that avoiding certain behaviors will decrease one's risk of heart disease greatly. Women already face high odds of acquiring problems with their hearts; why exacerbate the risks by indulging in avoidable behaviors? Though the question is a pointed one, the answer can be quite complicated.

For one, we could look at the lifestyle that modern women lead. Though I believe stress levels have not changed, the types of stress have. Secondly, childhood experiences have a major impact. If one's parents smoked or ate a certain diet or led sedentary lives, it is much more likely that one will adopt the same habits. It takes a great deal of energy, commitment, and consistency to change a long-ingrained habit learned in childhood. Finally, there are some risks we take that are simply unavoidable. Genetics and even fate play a large part in how our bodies will age and what diseases they will or will not acquire.

In many ways, we have become a risk-averse society. In the summer, as a child, I played outside with friends all day. We had a certain freedom and responsibility. Now, in many places, it is unthinkable to let children play outside unattended. We wear a seatbelt and helmets, actions that were exceptionally rare just twenty years ago. Most new parents baby-proof their homes, while in my day it was likely that a child learned about electrical outlets by the old "try it and you won't like it" method.

The early American Indians did not stop a child from rushing toward an open campfire. They were allowed to be burned as a means to learn quickly about the dangers and pain that come with fire.

In my youth, a friend of mine fell from a jungle gym at school and broke his arm. Then it was considered an accident, and you can bet he was more careful the next time he tangled with the jungle gym. Now, the school and supervising teachers run a good chance of being sued for negligence for allowing children to play on dangerous equipment.

How is it that we have become so completely safety-conscious and yet so reckless with our own health, our most precious commodity? Why is it that we protect ourselves from germs by buying special antibacterial everything but smoke cigarettes that will permanently damage our lungs? A person that would never get on a bike without a helmet might end up avoiding exercise at all because it is "inconvenient." A parent that would never allow their child to talk to a stranger stops for a fast-food lunch without considering the impact on their nutrition, let alone the cholesterol content of a greasy hamburger and fries.

Consequences

If we are to be responsible for our future health, the most important thing is to understand the cumulative impact of our daily actions (or inactions). What seem like minor points today may accumulate over the years and become a major issue. Is one cigarette going to blacken your lungs irreparably? No. Is one hamburger going to laden your arteries with plaque? No. Is one day without an adequate amount of movement going to weaken your heart? No. But months and years of such activities will.

There are over 200 potential individual risk factors for heart disease, but don't let the "odds" overwhelm you. The top three—high cholesterol, high blood pressure, and smoking—can, in most cases, be prevented. We will discuss many ways that you can improve your health and at the same time lessen your risk factors.

We are going to take a look at the risk factors for heart disease with specific respect to women. There are many that are unique to women. While you are reading through this information, keep a running dialogue with yourself about your own sense of risk and about what habits are constructive and what habits aren't. Keep a rough mental tally of your overall risk and where you fit on the continuum of health. And while you are making this evaluation, consider not only yourself but other young women as well. Even though it may not be evident at first, by mitigating your own risks through healthy choices, you will be influencing other women, perhaps even your own daughters, to undertake the same choices, and you will be leading them toward a full life of full health.

Diabetes

According to the American Heart Association, a woman with diabetes mellitus is five to seven times more likely to develop heart disease or have a heart attack or stroke, whereas a man with diabetes is only three to five times as likely. Diabetes is a complicated illness because it opens the door for other illnesses, along with the fact that many precursors for heart disease are also precursors for diabetes. For example, women with diabetes also often have high cholesterol, are overweight, and have high blood pressure.

There are two general types of diabetes and several subsets. Type-1 diabetes is known as juvenile-onset diabetes. Its onset typically happens in infancy and childhood. It occurs when the body's immune system attacks and destroys the cells in the pancreas that create insulin. This type of diabetes always requires insulin. At this time, little can be done to prevent it.

Over 9 million women in the United States have Type-2 diabetes, and this is the type that concerns us most. It can begin as "insulin resistance," meaning the body cannot use insulin properly, and eventually leads to severe diabetes that must be controlled with insulin injections. In the past, this was primarily a disease of older age, but it is increasingly being diagnosed in young children as well.

Did You Know?
The total costs of Type-2 diabetes related to obesity in 2001 totalled nearly $98 billion.

Type-2 diabetes, for the most part, is preventable and controllable. I believe the increasing numbers have roots in the changing diet and activity levels so common in our modern lifestyle. Today, physical activity is something that we must seek out, plan for, and schedule. In days past, physical activity was a matter of everyday survival. Our diets are high in carbohydrates and refined sugar. Only a few hundred years ago, sugar was an expensive treat to be had only on very special occasions. Our bodies simply are not designed to handle the amounts of refined foods that we eat today. Sugar, when it is present in the blood in excess amounts, has the ability to scratch the inner lining of our blood vessels. These small scratches can eventually lead to atherosclerosis—a concept we will discuss in depth later in the book.

If you have a genetic predisposition to diabetes—for example, having a near relative who also has diabetes—then it is especially important for you to reduce your risk. A genetic link does not spell a certain diagnosis. Leading a healthy lifestyle will go miles toward reducing the possibility that you will develop diabetes.

Of special concern for women is diet during pregnancy. It is especially important to eat healthy foods and avoid refined sugars. A woman that develops gestational diabetes has a 25-50% greater chance of developing diabetes within 5 years, not to mention the risks of having a large baby and other complications.

HEALTHY STEPS

- ♥ Nutritious diet
- ♥ Moderate exercise
- ♥ Fasting glucose blood level once a year

Obesity

Over the centuries, women's waistlines have fluctuated with fashion trends, just like hemlines. There have been periods of time where it was considered "sexy" to be full-figured. In our modern times, the sought-after figure is dangerously thin. Given that women feel pressure to meet unrealistic expectations of maintaining a stick-thin figure, why, as a population, are we becoming heavier than ever? In 2001, nearly 21% of the population was considered obese, a 75% increase from 1991. This belies the fashion trend toward being model thin. Women, it seems, have become trapped by unrealistic expectations that have led to a backlash of sorts. This backlash is costing them their health and their peace of mind.

Obesity is a risk factor

You Diagnose It

Ann presented to my office at the age of forty-two. Her main concern was that she was becoming increasingly short of breath with any type of activity at all. Over the past few months, it had become difficult for her to walk even a few yards without feeling "out of breath." She had also noticed some swelling in her ankles. Upon further questioning, she admitted to using three pillows to sleep at night but didn't really think anything of it until I asked about it specifically.

Upon examination, I found her to be 5 feet 4 inches tall and 440 pounds. Her pulse was about 100 beats per minute and her blood pressure was 140/90.

What do you think might have been causing Ann's sudden shortness of breath? If you were in Ann's position, what would you expect from your cardiologist in terms of treatment and/or advice?

Discussion

In cases of morbid obesity, such as Ann's case, the heart simply cannot keep up with the demands the body places on it; the medical terminology is cardiac overload. It was difficult to come to a complete diagnosis because her weight precluded the ability to do an exercise stress test. Her size also exceeded the safety limits for cardiac catheterization equipment.

When she first visited me, the best I could offer was a medication to control her high blood pressure and diuretic drugs to help rid her of fluids being stored in her tissues because her heart was not able to move them out effectively. The only real "cure" was weight loss. I offered her a medically-managed diet and physical therapy. The physical therapy was useful because it allowed her to attain some physical movement under the watchful eye of a professional. She was able to gradually increase her activity as her tolerance increased, and her weight has since dropped.

Obesity, in and of itself, is enough to cause severe cardiac difficulty. Even moderate weight loss can be enough to improve heart function and relieve symptoms of heart failure.

---

not only for diabetes, but also for heart disease and a host of other undesirable health complications. Obesity slows recovery from illness and injury. Fat cells themselves are responsible for storing and releasing harmful chemicals. Obesity also hinders daily life. It affects tolerance of physical activity, feelings of well-being, self-image, and emotional health. If you are already struggling with obesity, you don't need me to tell you that it can impact your intimate relationships and even your relationships with your children.

According to an article in the *Wall Street Journal* in March 2002, "A study of 575 otherwise healthy young women found that 25% had abnormally large hearts. More disturbing, 20% of the women in the study were diagnosed with left ventricular hypertrophy, an enlargement of the heart's main pumping chamber—and a condition highly predictive of future heart problems. Nearly all of the women with the condition were obese; the average age of the group was twenty. Dr. Kimball says that he and his colleagues at Cincinnati Children's Hospital are studying a younger group of children and are finding that abnormalities in hearts of obese children begin to form in the early teens or even sooner."

Clearly, this is not just an issue of middle age. The foundations of health and diet begin in childhood, and we are failing our children. We are failing to educate; but more importantly, we are failing to provide a healthy example. The outcome of this is an increasingly overweight society, skyrocketing medical costs, and untold increases in the numbers of chronic illnesses.

Obesity is a precursor to diabetes, a potentially devastating illness we have already discussed. The vast majority of overweight women will also have elevated blood pressure, which we will discuss later in this chapter. Fat tissue actually produces substances that increase blood pressure. Every 10 pounds of fat produces an equivalent of 10 mg of cholesterol per day, regardless of dietary intake. Worst of all, experts believe that every extra one pound of body weight subtracts one month from overall life expectancy.

The statistics are frightening, and the reality is deadly. Obesity is a condition I liken to cancer. It is invading our society, and the reasons are deeper and more complicated than scientific medicine is equipped to provide. Food, as we know it in modern society, often symbolizes so much more than something we eat to satisfy our physical requirements. We must find a way to incorporate food into our daily lives as a fact of life rather than using it as a dysfunctional focus.

The Numbers

- Nearly 2/3 of adults in the United States are overweight, including 64.5 million women (61.9%).
- Nearly 1/3 are obese, or 34.7 million women (33.4%).
- Medical spending due to overweight and obesity was $92.6 billion in 2002 dollars.
- Americans spend an average of $33 billion every year on weight loss drugs, programs, and other aids.

(Numbers courtesy of the National Institute of Health)

HEALTHY STEPS

- ♥ Eating for health, not emotional comfort
- ♥ Daily movement and activity
- ♥ Social connections

Abnormal Lipids/High Cholesterol

You probably don't need a lecture from me on cholesterol. We have all been well educated on the importance of keeping your cholesterol numbers under control. In fact, low numbers are now thrown around almost like a badge of honor. It is important to look through the "trendiness," the media hype, and the drug manufacturers' advertising and realize that cholesterol levels do have a major impact on future heart disease. We will discuss, in great detail, the process of cholesterol building in the blood and how this condition can escalate to a serious problem, but it also deserves a mention in this chapter.

High cholesterol levels actually lay the groundwork for coronary artery disease, in the form of atherosclerosis. These conditions impact your heart by either cutting off circulation, by occluding arteries and veins, or by "blowing off" the lining of your vessels and forming clots elsewhere in the body. This can lead to a stroke or a heart attack depending on where the clot lodges.

Fat in the blood comes in two basic types: cholesterol and triglycerides. As these fats travel through our blood stream, they attach themselves to proteins. This new "package" is called a lipoprotein, of which there are some basic types we concern ourselves with: high-density lipoprotein (HDL), low-density lipoprotein (LDL), and lipoprotein a (LPa). The National Institutes of Health

New Discoveries

Increasing activity and adjusting diet really do reduce the other risk factors for heart disease. In this study, there were 120 women who were premenopausal and clinically obese. These women did not have diabetes, hypertension, or high cholesterol levels when they began the study.

The women modified their diets to one similar to the Mediterranean diet we outline in this book and increased their activity, mainly through walking and swimming. After two years, their body-mass index decreased, which was expected. More importantly, they had lower levels of the inflammatory markers that doctors look at as potential risk factors for heart disease or heart attack. (Esposito et al. 2003)

(NIH) has provided guidelines for target cholesterol levels. Everyone should strive to meet these standards, women and men alike.

- ♥ HDL is often referred to as "good" cholesterol. It removes excess cholesterol from the system. This number should be higher than 60. If it is less than 40, it is considered a major risk factor.
- ♥ LDL is referred to as the "bad" cholesterol. It builds up on the lining of the vessels and becomes plaque. This number should be less than 100. Anything over 130 is considered high.
- ♥ LP(a) is a relatively newly-discovered lipoprotein. It carries a protein that may impair the body's ability to dissolve clots. It is being investi-

gated as a risk factor for coronary disease. This is not routinely tested for yet.

♥ Triglycerides are actually fatty acids, which are the basic chemicals found in fats in both animals and plants. Less than 200 is optimal.

Healthy Fat

Fat, fat, fat. It is everywhere. In our food, on our bodies. We are deathly afraid of it and fight a daily battle against it, yet we seem to be losing. Maybe it would help to understand that not all fat is bad—in fact, some of it is necessary. Here are some of the types of fats and their place in your diet:

Saturated Fats and Cholesterol: These fats are typically of animal origin: meat, dairy, and eggs. Saturated fats are a great source of calories, and cholesterol is vital to the body for producing certain hormones. These fats are "natural," but they are also solid at body temperature. Our bodies typically produce enough cholesterol, without receiving it via diet, to meet its needs.

Unsaturated Fats: These fats are typically of vegetable origin. They include seed and vegetable oils. We must all have a certain amount of unsaturated fatty acids to live. The best of these are the omega-3 and omega-6 fatty acids found in cold-water fish. Our bodies are not capable of creating omega-3 or omega-6 fatty acids; therefore, it is important to get them through diet. Good sources are extra virgin olive oil, flax seed, sunflower seeds, and pumpkin seeds. All oils are damaged by heat and light and can produce trans fats. Therefore, is best to cook with clarified butter or tropical oils. Extra-virgin olive oil is a readily available choice and does not degrade as much as other vegetable oils.

Trans Fats: If you want to point a finger at a big, bad fat, this would be the one. Trans fats do not occur in nature and they derive entirely of unsaturated oils that have been heated to produce a long-lived, very stable fat. These types of fats are found in many processed foods and can wreak all kinds of havoc on your body. They are known to increase cholesterol levels by a larger percentage than other fats, raise lipoprotein a, lower the efficiency of the immune system, decrease insulin response, and increase the rate of cancer death. These fats are "manufactured" simply for the purpose of extending shelf life and improving texture or taste—small benefits for such incredible drawbacks.

These numbers should provide target goals as well as a starting point for discussions between you and your health-care provider. There will be variability from person to person, and the ratios will also be different. It is especially important to go over your cholesterol levels with your physician and get his or her input on how best to manage your risk.

It is also important to bear in mind that cholesterol does not come just from fatty foods. You can have a genetic predisposition to higher levels of cholesterol. If this is the case, it is very important to be tested in your 20s and be tested often. It would also be wise to have a discussion with your

doctor about aggressive strategies for keeping your numbers in check.

HEALTHY STEPS

- ♥ Proper nutrition and diet. Avoid trans fatty acids and incorporate "healthy" fats into your diet.
- ♥ Move, move, move. Keep the blood flowing and your body systems equalized.
- ♥ Get your cholesterol level checked. If the numbers are okay, check them again in five years. If they are elevated, discuss methods for lowering your cholesterol with your physician.

Family History

The nature-versus-nurture argument has been an ongoing one throughout medical history. It is one of the founding quandaries of all research. Unfortunately, the jury is still out on the topic. It is my guess that eventually the truth will be in the middle. I certainly believe this to be the case with heart disease.

A study published in *Circulation* in January 2001 found that people with a first-degree relative with heart disease, even if they had no other risk factors or symptoms, had a 50% greater chance of showing atherosclerosis on a PET scan. (Sdringola et al. 2001)

It seems that the highest risk is if you have a close relative that developed heart disease at a young age, under fifty for a father or brother and under sixty for a mother or sister. When that is the case, you have a 25% to 50% chance of developing the same level of disease at the same age. As we discuss elsewhere in this book, family history is not a death sentence. It is merely one factor out of many that can lay the groundwork for developing an illness.

Table 3.1

Family History of CHD and Stroke in Health Family Tree Study

Family History Score[b]	% Families	% Early Disease	% All Disease
CHD			
≥0.5	14	72	48
≥1.0	3.2	35	18
≥2.0	1.0	17	6
Stroke			
≥0.5	11	86	68
≥1.0	1.4	22	16
≥2.0	1.0	19	12

[a] Includes data from 122,155 families; 16,602 early CHD cases; 54,182 cases of CHD at any age; 4600 early stroke cases; and 22,425 cases of stroke at any age.

[b] Family history calculated using events in families at time of data collection (1983-1999). Family History Score (FHS) defined by comparing the number of CHD events (heart attack requiring hospitalization, coronary bypass surgery, or percutaneous angioplasty) in a family to the expected number of events based on the age and sex of family members and population incidence rates; FHS >1.0 requires having at least two affected persons at any age in the family.

Note: Adapted from Williams et al.

CHD, coronary heart disease. (Hunt et al. 2003)

In the case of heart disease, you must take precautions such as not smoking, exercising, and eating healthfully. All of this will do wonders for reducing your risk, regardless of your family history. When you and your physician are assessing your own personal risk, family history will weigh heavily, but so will other preventive steps.

HEALTHY STEPS

- ♥ Interview family members to determine the extent of heart disease in your family.
- ♥ If you have a first-degree relative with heart disease, keep a close eye on your blood pressure and cholesterol. Consider keeping a blood-pressure cuff at home and talk with your doctor about how often to have your cholesterol checked (once per year, minimum).
- ♥ Take as many preventive measures as possible to tip the scale in your direction.

Hypertension

High blood pressure is a condition to which most people in the modern world can relate. I'm sure we have all at one time or another felt our blood pressure rise. Maybe when you're stuck in traffic or someone cuts you off, maybe the boss is yelling at you or the kids just won't settle down. Maybe your husband is angry with you or you have had an argument with your best friend. Any one of these situations is enough to set a woman's survival instincts into high gear and kick the blood pressure up.

In Juanita's Words

I was thirty-four, a new mom, and tired all the time. I had left my job to stay home with our new baby, but I was still stressed. I know I wasn't sleeping enough. Who ever does with a newborn in the house? One day, on a whim, I checked my blood pressure on the machine at the pharmacy. The reading said 150/90. Needless to say, I was surprised and got checked out by the doctor. Their reading came in at 140/90. Not dangerously high but still in the elevated category. My doctor says it will be manageable with some modest diet and lifestyle changes. I'm glad we caught it before any real damage was done.

Blood pressure is an amazing process used by the body for many different purposes. It can signal health or extreme disease. High blood pressure can be helpful or detrimental. Because the body often uses high blood pressure for a specific purpose and it is a natural state, the body does not always react to it in ways that let you know what is going on. That is why it has come to be known as the "silent killer." Most people can have excessive hypertension for years and not know it.

Though there may be times when your body requires high blood pressure, as in a fight-or-flight situation, it can be too much of a good thing. Imagine a thin rubber tube with water pulsing through it. If the tube is the proper diameter and the volume of water is just right, the water will flow freely with little impact on the tube itself. However, if one were to clamp down on the tube or the water vol-

---

DASH Diet

The DASH diet is a longstanding and respected diet prescribed frequently for patients with high blood pressure or congestive heart failure. It is based on increased servings of fruit and vegetables and decreased amounts of sodium. It is not a weight-loss diet, as it is also based on 2000 calories per day. However, it is a healthy diet that greatly improves blood pressure levels. Here are the basics.

- Grains, 7-8 servings daily.
- Vegetables, 4-5 servings daily.
- Fruits, 4-5 servings daily.
- Low-fat or fat-free dairy foods, 2-3 servings daily.
- Meats, poultry, or fish, 2 or fewer servings daily.
- Nuts, seeds, and dry beans, 4-5 per week.
- Sweets 5 per week.

Sodium occurs in small amounts in natural foods, so it is essential you take in as few processed foods as possible; and of course, do not add any salt to foods you prepare. The diet aims for an intake of 1500-2400 mg a day. For more information, visit the website at **http://www.nhlbi.nih.gov/health/public/heart/hbp/dash/**

ume were to increase, the pressure exerted on the tube would be much greater. It would also take more force to pump the water through the tube. That, in a nutshell, is hypertension.

After a period of time, the vessels become injured and fatigued from accommodating a high pressure within their lining. This leads to atherosclerosis. It also makes the chance of a blood clot much greater, as the high pressure exerted on the plaque lining the vessels can tear a piece of plaque loose and set it free in the cardiovascular system, where eventually it will lodge, either in the a small vessel or in the brain, causing a stroke.

The heart also becomes tired from working so hard to pump blood under high pressure conditions and develops thickened muscles. In the age of bodybuilding, this might sound like a good idea, but it is actually very damaging to the heart.

Hypertension can lead to problems with other organs. For example, the tiny vessels in the eyes are very sensitive and easily damaged, as are the vessels in the kidneys. Hypertension is one of the leading causes of kidney failure.

Luckily, blood pressure is easily checked and easily treated. Unless your blood pressure is incredibly high, your first steps to lowering it will involve diet and exercise. If these methods fail, there are many, many good medications on the market that will lower your blood pressure as well.

In May 2003, a new study released by the National Heart, Lung, and Blood Institute changed the guidelines for blood pressure. The new guidelines state that "normal" blood pressure is under 120 systolic (the top number) and 80 diastolic (the bottom number). 120-140 or 80-90 is considered pre-hypertension, and higher than 140 or 90 is hypertension. These numbers are considerably lower than the original guidelines used by doctors for years. Though somewhat controversial, the lower numbers, according to most doctors, will help physicians more quickly identify and work with patients who are at risk for developing hypertension later in life.

Table 3.2
Blood-Pressure Classifications

Category	Systolic	Diastolic	Lifestyle Modification
Normal	Less than 120	Less than 80	Encourage
Pre-hypertension	120-139	80-89	Yes
Stage 1	140-159	90-99	Yes
Stage 2	Greater than 160	Greater than 100	Yes

Blood pressure cuffs are inexpensive, and it is a simple matter to check your own blood pressure at home. If you find this isn't feasible, there are free blood-pressure machines at many pharmacies, and staff at fire stations will always check your blood pressure for free. There are no excuses for "not knowing."

HEALTHY STEPS

- ♥ One more time: Proper diet and activity.
- ♥ Decreased salt intake. Thirty percent of the population with hypertension have a sensitivity to salt, meaning salt intake affects their blood pressure in greater proportion than normal.
- ♥ Biannual blood pressure checks, more frequently if you have a history of high blood pressure.

Sarah's Story

The presentation went well, my boss missed the fact that I was late, and I managed to sneak in past the receptionist so she won't be able to rat me out. The clients accepted the first proposal I offered, and the boss is all smiles. He invited me to lunch to talk about "incorporating" the client into our services, and I smell a raise, maybe even a promotion, coming my way.

As the room empties, I realize I'm exhausted. The entire left side of my jaw and neck hurts now. The stupid tooth is really annoying. I'm still sweating, and I think I need to eat something to settle my stomach. I'm never one to turn away a donut, but they don't really look good to me this morning. Could be I'm getting sick. Guess I better load up on some Vitamin C and Echinacea. Last I heard there was a nasty flu going around, and that's the last thing I need.

Of all the crazy things, my cell phone sputters a wet-sounding ring. I didn't think the darn thing would work, but it's making a valiant attempt. Caller-ID shows displays the number of my son's school. Can't be anything good. I answer with a hesitant-sounding "hello."

"Mrs. Sedaris?" The dreaded voice of Josh's principal.

"Yes. This is Sarah. We know each other well enough now, Mr. Staples. Call me Sarah."

"Okay, Sarah. I'm afraid we need you or your husband to come to the school to pick Josh up. I am sending him home for the day to consider his actions this morning."

"Great. What happened?" If it wasn't bad enough that my tooth was screaming in agony, now my head was working up its own heavy metal beat, to the tune of "Josh Is in Trouble Again."

"Well, it seems one of his classmates, Jeff Durante, let loose with a few choice names for Josh, and Josh let loose with a few punches and a kick for good measure. I'm sure it is no surprise to you that Josh has a temper, but we really need to stem his outbursts. I want him to take the day off to think about his anger, and then we can talk further about how to help him express himself differently. Can you pick him up within the next hour or so?"

"Actually, I can't. I will call my husband and send him over to pick Josh up."

"I will hold him here at the office until then. I'm sorry for the trouble, Sarah, but he is a good kid. We'll work it out with him. Please call tomorrow to set up a time to meet with me and Josh's counselor."

"Thanks. I will do that."

As upset as I am with Josh, I'm even more upset that I can't pick him up; but I don't dare miss the lunch meeting with my boss. It is just too important. I will have to call his father, and heaven only knows what he will have to say about it all. I'm sure he will try to contain himself, but my husband has a bit of old school in him. He will have a hard time hiding his pride in the fact that his son "stands up" for himself. Guilt notwithstanding, I simply don't have a choice today. I dial my husband's number and scrounge in my briefcase for some much-needed aspirin.

Sedentary Lifestyle

I will not go into depth on this topic here, as you will hear about it again and again throughout this book. Movement is absolutely critical to keeping your heart healthy. Instead, let me give you some facts and figures to consider.

- ♥ Nearly 300,000 people die each year from diseases and health conditions related to lack of movement and poor eating habits. This number is almost on par with deaths from smoking.
- ♥ These diseases add up approximately $117 billion annually in health care costs.
- ♥ 12. 6 million people have coronary heart disease, 1.1 million people suffer from a heart attack each year, nearly 17 million people have diabetes, and nearly 50 million adults are obese. Worse than that, the number of adolescents that are obese has tripled in the last twenty years.
- ♥ There is simply no way around it. Your health hinges on the amount of activity you undertake each day, and EVERY little bit counts. Don't underestimate the value of walking to the grocery store or taking the stairs.

What, exactly, are some of the benefits of physical activity?
- ♥ Activity pumps more blood through the veins, which increases the size of the arteries. This helps to prevent occlusion and diminishes the likelihood of a blood clot.
- ♥ Strengthens the heart muscle, which in turn decreases how hard your heart has to work to pump the same amount of blood. This reduces the risk of a heart attack.
- ♥ Increases "good" cholesterol and lowers total cholesterol.
- ♥ Lowers blood pressure.
- ♥ Lungs become better conditioned.

Stay With It!

There are many, many reasons to exercise, but just as many things distract us from our goal of daily activity. Here are some tips to staying motivated.

Look good: No one wants to worry about how they look when they are sweating and tired, but if you look good in your workout clothes, you will be more likely to show them off. Don't rely on grimy old t-shirts and worn sweatpants. Invest in some new yoga pants or a CoolMax shirt. Buy things that you WANT to put on.

Try a sport: Exercise comes in many forms. Recreational tennis, volleyball, and softball are all great forms of exercise, not to mention social occasions and a lot of fun.

Mix it up: Vary your exercise routine from day to day. You will gain health benefits and stay mentally and emotionally refreshed.

- ♥ Stimulates the natural process of angiogenesis. This is how the body creates tiny new blood vessels to bypass clogged or diseased vessels.
- ♥ Reverses atherosclerosis.

If thirty minutes a day can achieve benefits like that, why not?

Smoking

Not enough bad things can be said about smoking. I know you hear it on the news, in the media, and from everyone that is a nonsmoker, but it is still not enough. If you have never smoked, then add ten years to your life and skip to the next section. If you are smoking or have smoked, I don't have enough pages in this book to write about all the ill effects, so we will deal only with the risks to your heart.

Kicking the Habit
Visit the web site for the American Lung Association. They have a free program called Freedom from Smoking that is handled completely on line. Look them up at *http://www.lungusa.org/ffs*.

Given that nicotine is a drug so deadly that one drop of pure nicotine on your tongue can kill you, why would anyone want to smoke? Well, anyone who does smoke can tell you that it is an addiction. In fact, research shows that nicotine affects dopamine production in much the same manner that cocaine and heroin do. There are few addictions more powerful than smoking. Also, interestingly enough, a study published in December 1999 in *Nicotine and Tobacco Research* found that women have a harder time quitting smoking than men because they feel a much greater relief from withdrawal effects with every cigarette. Simply, smoking makes women "feel better" more so than men. The cards are definitely stacked against women smokers. (Eisenberg et al. 1999)

If we leave aside the issues of aging skin, harmful effects on unborn babies, and lung cancer, smoking DOUBLES the risk for developing heart disease. With heart disease already being the leading killer of women, do you really want to double your risk?

What effects does smoking have on your cardiovascular system?
- ♥ It slows the transfer of oxygen from the blood to the body.
- ♥ It increases the heart rate by 15-25 beats per minute.
- ♥ Blood pressure goes up by 15-25 points.

And these are just the readily distinguishable impacts. Cigarette smoking has also recently become known to elevate the levels of fibrinogen, C-reactive protein, and homocysteine. These are three new risk factors for heart disease that we will be talking about a bit later. Smoking more cigarettes daily elevates these levels even further.

Should the worst happen and you suffer a heart attack? Continuing to smoke afterward increases risk of a second heart attack by 1.51 times. If you need to have angioplasty or some other procedure to open up blocked arteries, continuing to smoke will practically negate the benefits of the surgery.

If all of this isn't enough, smoking increases your risk of stroke by four times, and if you are taking birth-control pills, smoking increases your risk of heart disease by six to ten times.

There is just no way to skirt the issue. Smoking is an obvious and serious health threat. But much like an addiction to any drug, it is not easily dealt with. There may be a complicated emotional foundation to the addiction as well as the physical and chemical components.

There are many, many valuable and useful smoking-cessation programs available. We list several resources in the appendix of the book. Also, be certain to speak with your physician, who will also have recommendations. You can also discuss a combination patch/antidepressant therapy that many are now finding very effective.

HEALTHY STEPS

- ♥ Seek support in whatever form works for you—friends, family, groups, or professionals.
- ♥ Utilize their help to STOP smoking. Do it for yourself, because you deserve a healthier life.

Sleep Apnea

Obstructive sleep apnea raises the risk of heart disease by five times. Although more prevalent in men, 9% of women have this condition, and it is an important factor to consider. Studies have shown that post-menopausal women who are not on hormone-replacement therapy have similar rates of sleep-related breathing disorders as men. The good news is that, when treated, the risk of developing heart disease falls to almost zero.

> **Sleep: Too Much or Too Little**
> A study of 72,000 nurses published in the Archives of Internal Medicine reached some interesting conclusions about the importance of sleep. The study revealed that women with five hours of sleep or less a night were 39% more likely to develop heart disease than the women who slept for eight hours. On the flip side, women who slept an average of more than nine hours a night were 37% more likely to develop heart disease. The long-held belief in a solid eight hours a night still seems to be relevant. Strive for balance in everything, including sleep. (Avas et al. 2003)

Basically, sleep apnea is caused by an obstruction in the airway, either enlarged tonsils, enlarged adenoids, or fat tissue. This blockage causes a sleeping person to stop breathing and the oxygen level in their body to drop. When that happens, the body signals an alarm and wakes itself up in order to restore breathing. This constant wake-sleep pattern is unhealthy for a variety of reasons, including the problems that come with being excessively sleepy during the day, but also leads to the very serious potential of developing heart disease.

It can be difficult to determine if you have sleep apnea, but here are some signs to watch for:

- ♥ Waking up feeling groggy, tired, and wanting more sleep.
- ♥ Moderate to loud snoring, although it can be mild in some women.
- ♥ Pauses in breathing. Have your significant other observe your breathing patterns. Pauses may range from ten to sixty seconds or longer.
- ♥ "Snorts" upon resumption of breathing, often accompanied by movement in bed.
- ♥ Daytime tiredness, especially during quiet activities such as driving a car, working in front of a computer screen, sitting quietly (especially after a meal), reading, or watching TV.
- ♥ Frequent waking, especially to use the bathroom.
- ♥ Restless sleep.
- ♥ Morning headaches. Lack of oxygen during sleep can cause a serious headache.
- ♥ Lack of energy or feeling tired all the time.

There can be other causes for these symptoms, but if you experience several of them, it would be best to seek an evaluation by your doctor. Mention your suspicion about sleep apnea. There are take-home monitors that

What Is CPAP?

CPAP stands for Continuous Positive Airway Pressure. A CPAP machine is a piece of equipment that provides a continuous flow of air through a mask. This continuous flow is gentle but enough to keep the airway completely open, therefore preventing obstruction or snoring. This process mitigates the hazards associated with obstructive sleep apnea and the correlating heart issues.

are available now to gauge your breathing patterns during sleep. Some people simply set up a video camera that films them sleeping to look for signs of obstructed breathing patterns. Of course, if you have an alert sleeping partner, they may be able to make the diagnosis without any testing at all.

Sleep apnea can be treated by mechanical means, such as a CPAP (continuous positive airway pressure) machine. There are also surgical options available to remove the extra tissues blocking the airway. Losing weight is a good first step and may cure the problem entirely.

HEALTHY STEPS

- ♥ Interview your sleeping partner and ask specifically about signs of sleep apnea.
- ♥ Take a personal inventory of your quality of sleep. Do you feel your sleep is restful?
- ♥ Lose weight if necessary. Being overweight is the number-one cause for sleep apnea.
- ♥ Avoid drinking alcohol or taking sleeping pills. These drugs increase the occurrence of sleep-related breathing problems.

Oral Contraceptives

The link between heart disease and oral contraceptives is still relatively unexplored. There are a few known risks but still much more to learn, especially in light of the recent Women's Health Institute (WHI) study that we will talk about in the chapter on hormone-replacement therapy. At this time, it seems that oral contraceptives do NOT increase the risk of heart attack or stroke in women that are younger than thirty-five, as long as they don't smoke or have high blood pressure. In my mind, this link needs to be explored more fully. Let's talk about what we do know.

♥ Some birth-control pills may raise cholesterol levels and blood pressure.

♥ If you take birth-control pills and smoke, you GREATLY increase your chances of having a heart attack or stroke.

♥ If you have high blood pressure and use birth control, you increase your chances of a stroke by ten to fifteen times.

♥ The risk of developing a blood clot is three to four times higher than in women who do not take the pill.

♥ The increased risks for high blood pressure, heart attack, and stroke go down when you stop taking oral contraceptives.

Table 3.3
Alternate Methods of Birth Control

Type	Pros	Cons
Condoms for men	Good protection against STDs Readily available without a prescription	About a 95% effectiveness rate Noticeable during sex
Female condoms	Good protection against STDs Readily available without a prescription Does not reduce male partner's stimulation	A 79% to 95% effectiveness rate Noticeable during sex Can be difficult to insert Three times more expensive than male condoms
Spermicide	Available over the counter and inexpensive Enhances the effectiveness of condoms	Minimal protection against STDs Possible allergic irritation Questionable effectiveness when used alone
Diaphragm/Cervical cap	May be inserted before intercourse Some protection against STDs	Diaphragm is 80% effective Cervical cap is 60% to 80% effective Small risk of toxic shock syndrome Risk of allergic irritation
Injections	99.7% effective Convenient. One injection every 3 months	No protection against STDs Some report significant side effects
Implants	Up to 99% effective Convenient. May last for up to 5 years May be used while breast-feeding	Minor surgical procedure at doctor's office Irregular or unpredictable bleeding or spotting No protection against STDs
IUDs	Up to 98% effective Convenient. Requires little or no maintenance	Increased menstrual flow and cramps No protection against STDs Possible to expel the IUD without noticing it
Female Sterilization	99.5% effective Allows for spontaneous intercourse	Risks of surgical procedure Not easily reversible
Natural Family Planning	No cost No side effects No hormones	No protection against STDs Required education and record keeping Abstinence at specified times of the cycle
Vasectomy	99.85% effective Allows for spontaneous intercourse	Risks of a surgical procedure Not easily reversible

As with hormone-replacement therapy, the decision as to whether or not oral contraceptives are the right choice for you can be difficult. The current thinking is that if you are under thirty-five, don't smoke, and don't have any other risk factors for heart disease, birth control should be safe for you. Only you and your doctor can make that decision.

HEALTHY STEPS

- ♥ Investigate alternate forms of birth control. Weigh the risks and advantages.
- ♥ Open a discussion with your healthcare provider about the best options available to you. Be sure to discuss risks of heart disease.

Alcohol and Substance Abuse

My dictum is: everything in moderation, and the same holds true for alcohol. Most recent studies show that moderate alcohol intake—one glass of wine a day—has a positive impact on heart health. European countries have known this for years and commonly incorporate wine into their meals.

However, as with any addiction, alcohol in excess wreaks havoc on the entire physical system, including the heart. Drug abuse is equally as toxic. Either can damage your heart irreparably. Women are even more susceptible than men to the deleterious effects because women's bodies contain a smaller amount of water than men's. Therefore, the concentration of alcohol in a woman's body will be much higher than a man's, even if weight differences are taken into consideration. It is similar to pouring a shot of alcohol into a smaller glass of water. The concentration of alcohol will be greater.

In addition, alcohol-dependence-related diseases progress more rapidly in women than they do in men. Where a man might be able to drink for twenty or thirty years before developing disease, it may take a woman only fifteen to twenty years.

Drugs, even legal over-the-counter drugs, when used in excess are also very damaging to the heart. Addiction, in any form, is debilitating both emotionally and physically. It tears apart families and hearts alike. Not enough can be said for taking responsibility and accepting help.

In terms of the physical dangers, let's take a look at some specific abuse-related injuries:

♥ Alcohol: Alcoholic cardiomyopathy, a weakening of the heart muscle, is common in long-term drinkers. Eventually, this condition leads to heart failure. In some it may progress quickly, and in others it may take longer, but once the disease process has started, it is very difficult to reverse.

> **What About Red Wine?**
> Over the past ten years or so, there have been many studies touting the benefits of moderate consumption of alcohol, particularly red wine. It appears that a modest intake can help decrease cholesterol levels and lessen the overall chance of heart disease. The actual process by which this happens is still unknown, though it appears the presence of antioxidants and flavonoids may be partially responsible, the final results are still out. At this time, the American Heart Association does not recommend the consumption of alcohol just to receive these benefits.

♥ Cocaine: Regardless of how cocaine is ingested—by injecting, snorting, or dissolving it—it is quickly absorbed into the bloodstream, shooting through the major systems of the body, and gives it an incredible energy boost. Overstimulation of the heart leads to arrhythmias and possible sudden cardiac death. The coronary arteries can narrow or collapse, again leading to sudden death. The carotid arteries are equally susceptible and may collapse and narrow. This may lead to a stroke.

What is an Aneurysm?
A brain aneurysm is a weak spot on the lining of a vessel in the brain. The vessel bulges at this spot, putting pressure on surrounding brain tissues. It is possible for this vessel to rupture, which can lead to many complications, and usually death.

The stimulation from cocaine increases blood pressure exponentially, and we have discussed the dangers that brings with it. Finally, cocaine use significantly increases the risk of an aneurysm, which when it ruptures is nearly always fatal.

♥ Heroin: Heroin is an offshoot of morphine, which is a narcotic painkiller. After an initial "rush," it produces a relaxed effect on the entire body and has the opposite effects of cocaine. It lowers the blood pressure and slows breathing and heart rate. This severely diminishes the amount of oxygen available to the body. Heroin overdose is very common and very deadly. Also, the slowed pulse can lead to the formation of blood clots, resulting in a heart attack or stroke. If heroin is injected, eventually the veins collapse around the injection sites. Once these veins have collapsed, there is no way to return them to normal function.

♥ Marijuana: Thought of as a benign drug in many circles, it carries the same risks as smoking. In fact, research has shown that those with heart disease are at a higher risk of a heart attack within one hour of smoking the drug.

You Diagnose It

Jessica presented to the emergency room at the age of thirty-six. I was the cardiologist on call, so I was asked to examine her for further diagnosis.

She had chest pain below her sternum that radiated into her left arm. She was certain that she'd had a heart attack, and at that point, I believed it highly likely. Se smoked two packs of cigarettes a day and occasionally snorted cocaine, which she had used twenty-four hours before seeing me.

Upon examination, I found her pulse to be about 100 beats per minute and regular. Her blood pressure was 150/90.

What do you think might have been causing Jessica's sudden chest pain? She had previously been healthy and had never experienced chest pain of this type before.

DISCUSSION

In this case, the obvious thing to examine first is the use of cocaine. Cocaine is known to cause high blood pressure, increased heart rate, vasoconstriction (contracting of blood vessels), and an increase in oxygen consumption by the heart tissues. On one hand, the heart is demanding more oxygen. On the other, it is receiving a decreased blood flow because the vessels are constricting. This in itself is enough to cause chest pain.

The duration of drug abuse of the dose taken does not help a cardiologist in predicting the risk of a heart involvement. To make matters worse, even patients that have healthy or normal coronary arteries can suffer a heart attack after using cocaine just one time. Even low doses of cocaine can cause heart spasms leading to heart attack. It is known, however, that prolonged use of cocaine does indeed damage the heart tissues.

In Jessica's case, subsequent EKG testing did show that she had suffered a heart attack. She spent a few days in the hospital recovering. Unfortunately, after she left the hospital, she did not return for follow-up care, and I have no way of knowing whether or not she was able to abstain from cocaine and what long-term effects she might have suffered.

♥ Designer Drugs: Designer drugs, such as Ecstasy, are prevalent on the streets and readily available to people of all ages. They have also become very popular. Research is still out on many of these drugs, and new drugs are coming along every day. We do know that Ecstasy raises the blood pressure and heart rate similarly to cocaine. I am sure in the next few years we will be hearing much more about deaths from these drugs, particularly involving heart attacks.

HEALTHY STEPS

♥ If you don't already drink, don't start just to achieve benefits for your heart. It is better to invest your time and energy in diet and exercise.

♥ If you have a substance-abuse problem of any kind, please accept responsibility and seek help in whatever form works best for you. Twelve-step programs help thousands of people each year. Others do better with inpatient treatment centers. Only you can make the decision to seek help.

♥ If you have substance abuse in your past, be sure to discuss the issue with your doctor. He or she needs this information in order to provide you with the best screening tests.

Polycystic Ovary Syndrome

Polycystic ovary syndrome (PCOS) is a disorder in the endocrine system resulting in hormonal imbalances. Women with PCOS often do not ovulate and/or have increased levels of androgens. Most importantly, insulin resistance seems to be a central factor. With this comes increased cholesterol levels, weight gain, and a higher body-mass index.

Researchers at the Mayo Clinic found that, for these reasons, women with PCOS are at significantly higher risk for heart disease. Some of the symptoms of PCOS are—

- ♥ Skipped periods
- ♥ Excess body hair
- ♥ Infertility
- ♥ Obesity, apple-shaped figure
- ♥ High blood-sugar levels

If you are diagnosed with PCOS, be certain to undergo thorough and regular screenings for heart health, including cholesterol and blood-pressure checks. The best steps you can take are to increase your exercise and follow a low-carbohydrate diet. Diet is especially important due to the insulin-resistance component of the syndrome.

HEALTHY STEPS

- ♥ Low-carbohydrate diet and plenty of activity
- ♥ Frequent blood-pressure and cholesterol-level checks

African-American/Hispanic Heritage

All women of color, regardless of racial and ethnic backgrounds, are at higher risk for heart disease. African-American women are 28% more likely to die of a heart attack and 78% more likely to die of a stroke. This is, in part, due to higher rates of diabetes, hypertension, and obesity. Hispanic women are not exempt from these frightening statistics.

Black Women at Risk

Black women are twice as likely as white women to have or die from coronary heart disease but are less likely to receive adequate treatment. (Weintraub and Vaccarino 2003)

Nearly 50% are overweight and sedentary and 17% have cholesterol levels that are considered too high.

The jury is still out on whether these increased numbers are a result of nature or nurture, but certainly we can speak to the numbers with respect to obesity and diabetes. These two risk factors alone are enough to cause increased numbers in heart disease.

Hispanic and black women need to be particularly alert to the dangers of heart disease and the risk factors leading up to it.

HEALTHY STEPS

- ♥ Increased awareness of heart disease and risk factors
- ♥ Community education about risk factors
- ♥ Healthy diet and exercise
- ♥ Frequent screenings as recommended by your physician

Sarah's Story

I survived the day only to stumble through the front door and land on the couch. I'm sure the kids are starving, but I feel terrible. My headache is still raging and my stomach is throwing in its two cents as well. I didn't eat at lunch, but at least a promotion seems imminent. I'm sure I must be coming down with something, because I've sweating bullets since the presentation this morning.

"Mom, are you home?" Josh is looking for me, and I'm not sure I want to answer him. I haven't decided how to talk with him about the fight at school earlier today. The guilty mom wins out.

"Yes, Josh. I'm here." I'm surprised at the resignation in my voice.

"Mom, I'm hungry." He bounds down the steps with his still little-boy lope and stops short of the couch. "Are you okay? You look terrible."

"Gosh son, thanks. By the way, you are in no position to place demands, and insulting me isn't going to do you much good, either. I want to talk with you about what happened today, but I just don't have the energy right now. Have your dad order a pizza and we will talk about this fighting thing after dinner."

"Mom, it wasn't my fault. You don't know what he was saying to me."

"Josh, I don't want to talk about it right now. We'll get into it later. Have your dad get the pizza and ask him if he'd come down to talk to me for a minute."

"Okay, Mom." His face displays a mixture of fear and defiance.

I'm sure the angry but courageous boy in him is warring with the little child that would like a hug from mom.

It takes so much strength to parent this little guy, and I love being a mom, but all I want right now is some sleep. My whole left side is aching and I think that just a few minutes of sleep would make all the difference.

"Sarah, are you looking for me?" That didn't take long. It would usually be hours before my husband would pull himself away from work to talk to me.

"Yeah. I was just hoping you would handle dinner. I'm not feeling well. I think I'm coming down with something." Again, the fatigue is obvious in my voice.

"I'm really busy trying to make a deadline, but you look awful. I'll handle it." And finally, the words I had been waiting for all day: "Why don't you go upstairs and get some rest?"

Diet Drugs

Women have so little support in life, particularly when it comes to their health. Too often they are forced to choose between caring for themselves and caring for others. Our culture does little to help. Women run an obstacle course, often not realizing their life depends on their health. They must avoid the purveyors of diet drugs that border on complete irresponsibility, the high-gloss magazines selling sex through images of women with ultra-thin bodies, and the sugar-laden and fatty foods that are so addictive. Where do women turn to when they are overwhelmed with responsibility and fatigued to the bone? In our fractured society, there is too seldom a trusted parental figure to turn to for seasoned advice or warmth. Their friends are likely mired in the same trap of stress and lack of nurturing. I often wonder: who is nurturing the nurturers?

When a woman is confronted with the need to

True Medical Story

A nurse at the beginning of the shift places her stethoscope on an elderly and slightly deaf female patient's chest wall. "Big breaths," instructed the nurse. "Yes, they used to be," sighed the patient.

lose weight, the stresses of life win out and too many women are lured to the promise of a "quick cure" for their weight problems in the form of diet drugs. I think most women understand there really is no quick cure. Diet and exercise need to be in line for real change to take effect. However, when faced with the choice between finishing a report for work or going to the gym for a quick work-out, work usually wins. When given an option between watching a child's soccer game or taking extra time shopping for healthy foods, the soccer game takes precedence. When it is six o'clock, you're just getting off work, and the kids are begging for dinner, fast food seems to be the reasonable option. No wonder the diet drug industry does over 39 BILLION dollars worth of business every year. Unfortunately, the majority of the available diet drugs are unsafe or ineffective.

Dangerous Drugs

The moment one drug is taken off the market because it has been found to be extremely dangerous, another rises up and takes its place. It seems that we are not willing to live without the hope that a pill can work magic. It is hard for us to hold to the fact that the weight is not the problem as much as the reasons behind the weight gain. Here is an example.

I had a patient several years ago—we'll call her Kate. She had lived most of her life with an excessive amount of weight, and it had truly shaped her self-image and confidence level. When she reached my office, she was thirty-one, obese, and dying of a valvular disease in her heart that had been caused by the use of the infamous diet drug fen-phen.

Here was a young woman who was beautiful and intelligent. She was successful in her work and had an active social life, yet she was so desperate to be rid of her excess weight that she was willing to close her eyes to the health risks. Most of you have probably heard of this drug. The amazing part of this story is that she purchased it on the black market AFTER the FDA had recalled it. She had heard of the drug, the health risks, and the lawsuits and still chose to use it in her effort to lose weight. She went on to have valve-replacement surgery but continues to experience shortness of breath when she is active.

Valvular Disease

The exact causes for valvular disease in fen-phen users are still unknown. Fen-phen is actually a combination of two drugs, fenfluramine and phentermine. In the women adversely affected by these drugs, physicians find a thickened appearance to the valves of the heart. This thickening is similar to the heart damage that occurs along with rare cancerous tumors that release serotonin into the bloodstream.

If all of this isn't bad enough, to add insult to injury, the average fen-phen user lost only 3% more weight than those that took a sugar pill! That is a lot of risk for very little benefit.

No End in Sight

With the huge outcry over the fen-phen side effects, one would think that diet drugs would lose their footing and that people would turn to other means of weight reduction, but in its place has risen another "wonder drug" that is equally dangerous, ephedra.

Ephedra is extracted from a natural herb called *ma-huang*. It has been known to cause toxicity and even death. It is known to cause high blood pressure, irregular heart rate, insomnia, nervousness, tremors, headaches, seizures, heart attacks, strokes, and even death. Despite this, people continue to take it in unsafe amounts. It is even more dangerous because it is touted as a natural drug, or "natural fen-phen."

Even the drugs prescribed by physicians have known side effects. Meridia is an appetite suppressant prescribed to those with a body-mass index greater than 30. Orlistat is also used to treat obesity by reducing fat

Trouble on the Internet

Do a quick internet search for just about any diet drug that you can name. Guaranteed, you will find many, many pharmacies willing to prescribe that drug for nothing more than a small consultation fee. In the cases of some overseas pharmacies, one only need provide a credit card number. Most of these pharmacies do not have your best interests in mind and are NOT looking out for your health. They are difficult to track down and difficult to regulate, which makes it difficult to hold them accountable. If you would like a prescription for a weight-loss medication, or any medication for that matter, it is best to be seen and evaluated by your physician first.

absorption. This drug is known to cause gastrointestinal upset. In both cases, patients must be monitored carefully for side effects. I don't recommend diet drugs in general, but I would NEVER suggest taking them outside of a physician's care. Even an innocent-sounding herb can have serious problems associated with it.

I do wish I had a magic pill, but I would rather it give women a fighting chance at improving their health, rather than artificially reducing their weight. I would rather you have permission to take the time to care for yourselves—shop for nourishing foods, eat in a way that is respectful to who you are, and find joy in movements that energize you.

Is it possible to take a diet drug and lose weight? Yes, of course it is. You can speed up your heart rate, pump your blood faster, increase the number of calories your burn, and decrease your appetite. But in the end, these are all just an artificial means to an end. The real secret is trusting yourself to find a path through life that makes sense to you, one that works for you, one that puts your health at the top of your priority list.

Taking a drug to lose weight is the first step on a slippery slope to an inaccurate body image and poor eating habits. I do believe there are genetically obese people that need medical assistance to gain a healthy weight, but I'm not sure diet drugs are the answer even in the most severe of cases. For the majority of women, it comes down to listening to your heart. It can tell you when it is stressed or healthy. It is asking you to respect it for the immense life force it is and use its capacity to make you healthier and stronger. It will pump as hard and as fast as you ask it to, whether that is through exercise or a diet drug. The heart is a wonderful organ that will expand to meet a challenge. It sustains marathon runners and casual walkers alike. It will bike for hundreds of miles or go sledding with the kids. It will do what you ask it to do if you take care of it. Use its strength and resilience without unnaturally stimulating it to excess. If you find yourself weighing the decision of whether or not to use a diet drug, even a seemingly innocent one, listen to your heart. It will make the right decision.

HEALTHY STEPS

- ♥ Find a source "diet buddy" or source of emotional support while adjusting your lifestyle.
- ♥ Become educated on a healthy diet and concentrate on long-term results rather than short-term gains.

Hormone-Replacement Therapy (HRT)

So that I don't repeat myself, we have an extensive chapter on hormone-replacement therapy later in the book that discusses of the pros and cons of undergoing estrogen replacement. There has recently been much controversy over whether or not HRT increases the risk of heart disease, and the latest studies show that to be the case. Please refer to the section on HRT and follow up with a discussion with your physician. This is an extremely important subject for women, and one that should not be taken lightly.

Stress

Our bodies still respond to stress as though we were cavemen living in a constant state of mortal danger. Over thousands of years, we have developed a response to danger, called flight or fight, that efficiently mobilizes our bodies to do exactly what they need to do to save us from a threat. Unfortunately for us, when we are being yelled at by the boss or are late for an appointment, our bodies interpret this much the same way it would if we were being chased down by a grizzly bear. The system works wonderfully if you have to use your leg muscles to outrun a charging rhino, but it breaks down with the constant use it gets in our daily lives.

Basically, your eyes and ears deliver information to your brain. The limbic systems, the part of our brains associated with emotion, interprets the information. If it sees a threat, it sends out a siren call. Once that happens, the hypothalamus kicks into action. It sends the message directly to the adrenal glands.

Chemicals, Chemicals, Chemicals

Our bodies contain complex mixtures of chemicals that rely on each other to perform their functions properly. Here a few that are used in the stress response.

Corticotrophin-releasing factor (CRF): Key regulator of the stress response. It is made and released by the hypothalamus, where it travels to the pituitary gland and signals the release of ACTH.

Adrenocorticotrophic hormone (ACTH): This is a hormone secreted by the pituitary gland. It stimulates the adrenal glands to produce cortisol and other hormones.

Cortisol: Cortisol is also known as the "stress hormone." It is a steroid hormone released by the adrenal glands. It reduces inflammation and mobilizes fatty acids and amino acids, as well as lowering blood-sugar levels. All of this contributes to our bodies being able to respond quickly in an "emergency."

Aldosterone: Also secreted by the adrenal glands under pressure from ACTH.

Thyrotropic-releasing factor (TRF): Again secreted by the pituitary gland to act on the pituitary gland.

Thyrotropic hormone (TTH): This is a hormone secreted by the pituitary gland to act on the thyroid gland. TTH stimulation cause the thyroid to release thyroxin.

Thyroxin: Thyroxin is responsible for increasing the basal metabolic rate, depth of respiration, heart rate and blood pressure, and anxiety. It also decreases feelings of tiredness.

They release adrenaline and noradrenaline. The hormones race through the bloodstream in order to kick start the body's organs. Second, the hypothalamus releases a chemical called corticotrophin releasing factor (CRF). CRF tells the pituitary gland about the imminent danger; it in turn releases ACTH. The ACTH, turned loose in the system, rushes to those by-now overworked adrenal glands and stimulates the release of a variety of chemicals, particularly cortisol and aldosterone. Cortisol stimulates the liver to release cholesterol, fat, protein, and glucose. It also steals energy from the immune system, effectively shutting it down. Aldosterone increases blood pressure so that your body can be ready on a moment's notice to take flight. This leaves behind a high sodium level in the blood, which attracts water and creates a great blood volume.

Stay with me—a lot is going on, and the body isn't finished yet. Third, the hypothalamus tickles the pituitary gland into releasing two more hormones, oxytocin and vasopressin. These hormones make certain that the blood pressure doesn't slack off and ramp up the body's ability to clot blood, just in case it happens to sustain an injury.

Finally, the hypothalamus, now exhausted, releases TRF. This also stimulates that overworked pituitary gland into releasing TTH. This hormone is responsible for telling the thyroid gland to produce thyroxin and triiodothyronine. These chemicals speed up metabolism. Blood pressure, breathing, heart rate, thinking processes, and perspiration all skyrocket, and the liver throws out more sugar into the blood to provide additional energy should your body need it.

Low Estrogen Levels in Young Women

A study published in 2003 in the *Journal of the American College of Cardiology* purported that young women with low estrogen levels may be at increased risk for coronary artery disease. Furthermore, they found that the lowered levels were a result of stress, leading to disturbed ovarian function and hormonal imbalances. (Bairey-Merz et al. 2003)

Now, that is a lot of work for your body to go through just because your neighbor is yelling at you for letting the dog into his yard. You may be mentally aware that the neighbor is not a threat, just a pain in the neck. However, your primitive limbic system doesn't know that. It perceives the stress as a threat and responds with its tried-and-true methods as if your life depended on it. The constant wear and tear on the body's systems, along with the elevated blood pressure, sugar levels, and other responses, leaves behind scars in the cardiovascular system. Worse yet, these responses happen on a very primitive level—and they happen automatically.

We are left with only a few choices. One, change your perceptions about what types of stressors are actually going to "stress" you. Two, develop a system of biofeedback you can use to keep your body systems in check when under stress. Both of these tasks are easier said than done, but with some diligence, they can be accomplished.

There are four key areas to examine: perception, control, coping, and personality style. Research has shown us that perception of stress is as important as the stress itself. Some women may perceive an impending deadline as stressful while other women thrive under the pressure. This is a matter of perception.

We also know that perceiving a sense of control plays a factor. Women who work in administrative positions with little influence over the course of their work are at a higher risk for heart attack than women in managerial positions.

Coping is closely linked to perception. We all cope with the stresses of life differently. However, research has found the most dangerous coping style is to repress feelings of anger or anxiety. Living in a sense of denial seems to send the limbic-response system into overdrive.

Finally, personality style plays a factor in stress response and long-term effects on the heart. A recent study done by researchers at Zion Women's Health Clinical Research Center found that "hostile" women with heart disease are twice as likely to have a heart attack or die from heart problems than women with a "milder" personality. The study found that hostility encompassing cynicism, anger, mistrust, and aggression played a large role in the long-term outcome of heart disease. (Chaput et al. 2002)

It will be up to you to assess your personality and your coping style. An honest evaluation is the key. Denying your pent-up anger or downplaying the impact of a stressful job will get you nowhere. Again, only you can best determine what you need to do to minimize the effects the stress in your life is having on your health. Some people chuck their busy lives altogether and seek out a simpler lifestyle. Others use formal biofeedback as a way to short-circuit the fight-or-flight response. For some, it is as simple as finding an outlet for their anxiety and energy; they take up a hobby or an enjoyable form of exercise.

Talk openly with yourself, your loved ones, and your healthcare team about the stresses you face on a daily basis. Assess yourself honestly and use your own intuition and others' input to stake out a plan that works for you.

HEALTHY STEPS

- ♥ Evaluate the current stressors in your life and map out a response plan.
- ♥ Seek out an activity, hobby, or friendship that will provide a source of release for anxiety and energy.
- ♥ Look for ways to establish a sense of control over your activities and destiny.

♥ Work on releasing hostilities and pent-up anger and responding appropriately to situations as they arise.

♥ Take whatever steps necessary to simplify your life toward a manageable, "de-stressed" level.

Depression and Antidepressants

There are many things to be thankful for living in our modern age. In the past, depression was regarded as a weakness or deficiency. Now, we know that often the root cause is chemical and there are many drugs available to combat the heavy weight and darkness depression creates. Psychoanalysis has made great strides in assisting people to ferret out emotional burdens that may be contributing as well.

It is also reasonable to assume that depression is a matter of the heart. We know that about one-fifth of people that have had heart attacks also suffer from major depression. Those with depression are three times more likely to die after a heart attack. There is clearly a correlation. When one feels depressed, it is often described as a weight in the center of the chest, or a heavy heart. There is still much to be learned about the link between heart disease and depression, or vice versa. Along with this, we have much to learn about the effects of antidepressant medications on the heart.

Depression can affect the heart rhythm, increase blood pressure, and alter the body's ability to clot blood. It also leads to elevated insulin and cholesterol levels. These symptoms, along with a low energy level and the inability to exercise, cause more than enough damage to the cardiovascular system. Factor in emotional pain, and the costs of depression are astronomical.

Gender Differences in Depression

1. Women have two to three times the rate of depression as men.
2. Women are threefold more likely than men to attempt suicide, yet two-thirds of completed suicides are men.
3. Atypical depression is a misnomer. It's actually the most common type of depression in women, who are more likely to report the atypical symptoms of oversleeping and overeating as part of their depression.
4. Depressed women have more psychiatric illnesses along with depression than depressed men.
5. Depression predisposes women with a history of alcoholism to alcoholic relapse.
6. Women account for 80% of cases of seasonal affective disorder.
7. Thyroid hormone, lithium, and stimulants appear to be more effective for augmentation of conventional antidepressant medications in women than in men.
8. Women are susceptible to one important type of adverse drug-drug interaction that men don't face—that between oral contraceptives and antidepressants.
9. Pre-menopausal women respond more quickly to SSRIs than tricyclic antidepressants. The opposite is true for men.

From Internal Medicine News, March 13, 2003," Gender Differences in Depression Response," by Bruce Jancin

Despite our modern treatment modalities, depression often goes unrecognized and/or untreated. For many, there is still a stigma attached to depression and seeking help for "emotional problems." Even if one does manage to find help for their depression, the choice of medications can be dizzying and confusing.

The older generation of antidepressants, known as tricyclics, has been linked to increased rates of heart disease. However, there is a growing body of evidence that the newer class of drugs, known as SSRIs, are actually effective at staving off worsening heart disease in those already struggling with it. They are known to reduce "platelet clumping," which in turns lessens the likelihood of clotting.

We also know that people suffering from depression have a difficult time fighting inflammation and carry higher levels of C-reactive protein. As you will read in a later discussion, this greatly increases the risk of suffering a heart attack.

Research on depression and antidepressant medication is evolving rapidly. Much, much more information will become available in the next few years. However, the general consensus at this point is that those suffering from depression should definitely seek help, either in the form of therapy or medication. If medication is the chosen route, the new SSRI drugs may do more than combat depression—they may improve your chances of staving off a heart attack.

The interplay of the mind-body connection with respect to depression is still quite a mystery, and there is much work to be done. However, it is not necessary to suffer with depression. Our current treatments have proven safe and beneficial, and with millions of people currently and successfully taking antidepressants, I think it is safe to say the stigma has been overcome.

HEALTHY STEPS

- ♥ Seek professional assistance if you suffer from depression. It is important to receive a trustworthy diagnosis.
- ♥ Discuss options for treatment. At this point, a combination of verbal therapy and antidepressant medications is the most effective.
- ♥ Find something enjoyable to do, even if it is a struggle at first. A hobby or enjoyable activity done on a regular basis will help to stimulate depression-fighting chemicals in the brain.

Pregnancy/Motherhood

Pregnancy and motherhood, being unique to women, earn a special place in the discussion about heart disease. Though one would never want to associate something as wonderful as pregnancy with a disease of the heart, there are some risks. Never would I suggest for a moment that this should deter one from bearing children. It is merely important to be educated about the facts so that you can guide your healthcare toward the best end possible.

Different Terms, Same Meaning
Pre-eclampsia
Pregnancy-induced hypertension
Gestational hypertension
Toxemia

Pregnancy carries with it some unique risks for the heart. The first and most common is pre-eclampsia, or gestational hypertension. This is basically the result of increased blood pressure during pregnancy. In a few women, increased blood pressure turns into pre-eclampsia, which can rapidly progress to a life-threatening state and warrants immediately delivery of the baby or, in the least, hospitalization under watchful care. Normally, the condition resolves with delivery of the baby. However, if you have had gestational hypertension, you are at increased risk of developing high blood pressure later in life and four times as likely to die of a stroke. If you had elevated blood pressure during pregnancy, it certainly warrants close observation throughout the course of your life.

The second condition that can affect your heart later in life is gestational diabetes. This is basically diabetes that comes on during pregnancy and, again, typically resolves with delivery of the baby, though a small percentage of women continue to have diabetes after giving birth.

Pregnancy after Heart Disease

If you have already had a diagnosis of heart disease, it is possible to carry a pregnancy to term. However, your pregnancy may be considered high risk, and you will need to be followed by a specialist, as well as your cardiologist. In the first trimester, the mother's blood volume increases by nearly 50%. This causes the heart to work harder in order to move blood through the system effectively. This change, along with others, can exacerbate pre-existing heart conditions. If you already have—

mitral stenosis, you may develop difficulty breathing, irregular heartbeat, and lung congestion. Medication may be required to regulate the heart rhythms. Intensive care is often required during labor and birth, with monitoring of the heart and pressures within the heart. After the birth, antibiotics may be prescribed to prevent endocarditis.

atrial septal defect, you will likely experience fatigue during pregnancy. However, more serious complications are rare.

ventricular septal defect, your heart may become more enlarged during pregnancy, but serious complications are rare.

aortic stenosis, you may be advised against becoming pregnant. Intensive care will likely be required, as well as antibiotic therapy following delivery.

mitral valve prolapse, a common heart defect in women of childbearing age, you may have a little difficulty during pregnancy. Antibiotics may be prescribed after delivery to prevent endocarditis.

Having gestational diabetes predisposes you to developing Type-2 diabetes later in life. If you had this condition during pregnancy, be certain to have your fasting blood-sugar levels checked at least once a year.

Researchers have also recently found that pregnancy, healthy and uncomplicated or not, reduces the amount of "good" cholesterol in a woman's body, and this drop persists for years. Having more than one pregnancy does not further push the HDL values down, but if you have other risk factors for heart disease, it would be wise to keep in mind.

Finally, there is a more serious condition called peripartum cardiomyopathy. This is a weakening of the heart muscle brought on during pregnancy. Occasionally—in about one out of every 10,000 pregnancies—a mother develops this condition. The signs and symptoms include shortness of breath and edema. The risk is greatest in women over thirty who have had previous pregnancies and in African-American women. Women who are pregnant with multiples also have an increased risk. Treatment includes medications to reduce fluid and regulate the heart rhythm. Within six months of delivery, 50-60% percent of women experience a complete recovery. But even if the problem is resolved, there is an increased risk of a recurrence with subsequent pregnancies.

Pregnancy-related heart problems have been known and researched for many years. However, researchers have now found that motherhood itself may be a risk factor for heart problems later in life. A ten-year study found that parenthood resulted in reduced leisure-time physical activities in women, but not in men. First-time moms seem to be the hardest hit. (Schmitz et al. 1999)

Additional children didn't impact the amount of time a woman spent undertaking physical activity. After becoming a mother, the women's activity levels dropped by 14%. Considering what we know about our already low levels of activity, a 14% drop can be disastrous. The study has not yet linked motherhood to actual incidence of heart disease, but it did draw a clear correlation to diminished activity levels. Anyone who has ever chased a toddler around the house might argue, but the major point remains. Exercise is critical to your heart health, and becoming a mother tends to rob women of the time they would normally spend doing exercise-directed activity.

HEALTHY STEPS

- ♥ If you are pregnant, good prenatal care is essential. The last three months of pregnancy are the critical weeks for watching for signs of heart difficulties or high blood pressure.
- ♥ If you have gestational diabetes or hypertension, make sure your physician is aware of it. They will guide you in getting the appropriate follow-through care.
- ♥ Use motherhood as a reason to be active, not an excuse to avoid activity. Incorporate your little one into your exercise routine, whether it be walking/jogging, bike-riding, or just romping in the park.
- ♥ If you had heart disease prior to becoming pregnant (see the sidebar), it may be necessary to have your cardiologist and a neonatal specialist follow your pregnancy.

Novel Risks

Research in cardiology has been making new discoveries by leaps and bounds in recent years, revealing a number of new or novel risk factors. Here are a few that you should know about. Though we are still learning about each of them, they are important enough to keep your eye on. They are considered novel risk factors because even though they seem predictive of future cardiac events, researchers are still uncertain whether treating them will reduce the likelihood of these events.

♥ **C-Reactive Protein:** This has been an exceptionally hot topic in cardiology research as of late. Recent studies have shown that CRP tests are almost twice as effective at predicting a person's risk for heart attack than are cholesterol levels. What is it exactly? Well, CRP is a marker for inflammation, which is the body's way of fighting an injury or infection. This inflammation seems to be present in the arteries of those with atherosclerosis years before they develop any serious symptoms. We are not yet sure exactly what causes low-grade inflammation, but we do know that it puts otherwise healthy people at risk. The latest research seems to suggest that an infection, possibly caused by a bacteria or virus, contributes to atherosclerosis. Scientists are now studying whether anti-viral medications can reduce the incidence of heart disease in people with elevated inflammatory markers, such as CRP. Currently, the best method we have for lowering CRP levels is the use of statins, the same class of drugs we use to lower cholesterol levels. These drugs seem to lessen the inflammation caused by atherosclerosis and decrease the amount of CRP found in the bloodstream.

> **CRP and Metabolic Syndrome**
> Data from the Women's Health Study shows that CRP levels taken in the context of Metabolic Syndrome, can further quantify the risk for heart disease. They were able to categorize women with Metabolic Syndrome into low-risk, medium-risk, and high-risk groups by examining the levels of CRP present in their blood. (Ridker etal, 2003)

♥ **Homocysteine:** In the late 1960s, a pathologist in Boston encountered two children with excessive homocysteine in their urine. They also had advanced atherosclerosis. At the time, he was ridiculed for suggesting a link between homocysteine and the formation of plaque on the artery walls. Today, however, we have shown a clear link between elevated homocysteine levels and coronary artery disease. Homocysteine is an amino acid formed during metabolism. The exact reasons for excess homocysteine are still unclear. Researchers are not sure if it causes coronary artery disease or if it is a result of it, but we do know that it can damage the arteries in a variety of ways. It can also affect the blood-clotting process. Like CRP, homocysteine levels can be tested.

Rheumatoid Arthritis and Heart Attack Risk

"Women with rheumatoid arthritis have a twofold higher risk of myocardial infarction than women without the autoimmune disease, according to evidence from the Nurses' Health Study."

Researchers suggest that if you have rheumatoid arthritis, you should keep a close eye on other risk factors, such as weight, cholesterol levels, diabetes, and family history. If you have significant risk factors in other areas, you and your physician might want to consider cholesterol-lowering drugs and blood-pressure medications, if necessary. (Ridker et al. 2003)

Currently, there is no solid research on ways to decrease the levels, though many are leaning toward a body of evidence that suggests vitamin-B deficiency may be a culprit and that augmenting a healthy diet with vitamin B can lower the presence of homocysteine.

♥ **LP(a)**: LP(a) is a lipoprotein with a chemical structure similar to "bad" cholesterol. Its presence has been linked to an increased risk, to that of three times normal, of heart attack. It is not a measure of inflammation, as CRP is, but an indication that inflammation is present. Most of the current treatments for lowering cholesterol do not lower the levels of LP(a).

♥ **Fibrinogen**: This is a protein synthesized by the liver that is necessary for proper blood clotting. However, its presence at elevated levels indicates a

---
Calcium Deposits Linked to CAD Risk

Researchers found that women with calcium deposits in the arteries of the breast were 20% more likely to develop coronary artery disease. These calcium deposits lead to arterial calcification, which can be detected by mammograms. This is yet another test to watch for in the future. (Waley 2002)

---

three-fold risk of developing cardiovascular disease. The higher the level, the higher the risk. Fibrinogen levels can be elevated by obesity, smoking, and other factors. One interesting association is that those with extremely stressful lives tend to have higher fibrinogen levels. Like homocysteine, there is no proven treatment for reducing fibrinogen levels.

HEALTHY STEPS

♥ If you already have a congregation of risk factors for heart disease, it is advisable to speak with your physician about being tested for these novel factors.

Metabolic Syndrome X

The final risk factor we are going to look at is what I liken to a modern epidemic. Metabolic Syndrome X is actually a cluster of risk factors that appear in a percentage of the population, an ever-growing percentage. If you have Syndrome X, it increases your risk of having a heart attack by four to twenty times. The cluster of risk factors for Syndrome X includes—

- ♥ Elevated insulin levels
- ♥ Central obesity (heaviness around the middle)
- ♥ High levels of LDL and triglycerides
- ♥ Hypertension
- ♥ Type-2 diabetes

Syndrome X is also known as insulin-resistance syndrome, because insulin resistance is key in the development of this condition. Insulin resistance is often the result of a diet high in refined carbohydrates and sugars. As we discussed earlier, insulin resistance comes about when the body is less responsive to insulin, which causes the pancreas to release even more insulin. This leaves excess insulin roaming free in the bloodstream and looking for more food to digest, hence a perpetual cycle of hunger, eating, and excess insulin. Current estimates are that ten to thirty percent of the adult population have some form of insulin resistance.

Next in line behind insulin resistance are our old friends obesity and sedentary lifestyle. I know, I know. You have heard me repeat myself over and over—and you will continue to hear it throughout this book—but I just don't have any other way to say it. Being overweight and inactive are the two riskiest characteristics to have in terms of developing cardiovascular problems.

Quick Quiz: Do I Have Metabolic Syndrome?

You might have Metabolic Syndrome if you have at least three of the following symptoms:

1. A waistline of 35 inches or more (measured across the belly)
2. A blood pressure of 130/85 or higher
3. A triglyceride level above 150
4. A fasting blood-glucose greater than 100
5. An HDL level lower than 50

What are some of the signs of insulin resistance?

- ♥ Elevated insulin levels
- ♥ Type-2 diabetes
- ♥ Central obesity
- ♥ High cholesterol levels
- ♥ Low level of HDL, the good cholesterol

- ♥ High blood pressure
- ♥ High levels of uric acid in the blood
- ♥ Smaller size albumin (micro-albumin) protein in the urine
- ♥ High levels of blood factors that promote clotting, including fibrinogen

If you fear that you are on the growing list of Syndrome-X victims, a battery of blood tests should be ordered to accurately diagnose the condition. Also, there are two visibly distinguishable characteristics common to the syndrome.

- ♥ **Body girth:** Measure the girth of your stomach at the level of your belly button. A measurement of more than 88 cm or 35 inches indicates a high risk of diabetes and heart disease. You can also measure your hips and calculate the ratio between your waist and hip measurements. A healthy number would be less than 0.85.
- ♥ **Skin lesions:** Often, Syndrome X will manifest in a dark thickening of the skin, especially at the neck and body folds. This is an indicator of insulin resistance.

Another surprising fact about Syndrome X is that it can cause a heart attack, even if you are on what would be considered a healthy, low-fat diet. This is definitely an instance where it is important to distinguish between healthy and unhealthy fats. Low-fat diets are usually extremely high in refined carbohydrates and sugars—a sure signal to the pancreas to produce yet more insulin. Don't be lulled into a sense of confidence in your diet just because your fat consumption is low. This is no longer considered an appropriate indicator for a healthy diet.

What to Do about Syndrome X?

You have taken an important first step in purchasing and reading this book. Understanding the nature of your heart and some of the hows and whys of heart disease will motivate you to care for the organ central to your body and spirit.

Heart disease can be exceptionally complicated, but avoiding it is exceptionally simple. Follow the Mediterranean diet (as we will discuss later) and get the appropriate amounts of exercise. Mitigate stress and strive for a benevolent outlook on life. Those four steps, though simple to describe, can be difficult to execute. However, they are the keys to avoiding heart disease and living a long and productive life. Successfully implementing them in your life will eliminate weight gain, diabetes, insulin resistance, and a host of other ills that set your heart up for difficulties further down the road.

Metabolic Syndrome and Stroke
Women with Metabolic Syndrome are 2.2 times more likely to
have a stroke than women without metabolic syndrome.

If you don't yet have heart disease or metabolic syndrome, now is the time to begin managing these risks and step forward into new, healthy habits. If you have already been diagnosed with heart disease, the good news for you is that it is never to late to halt it in its tracks and even, potentially, reverse it.

In the age of modern medicine, access to a variety of healthy foods, myriad options for enjoyable physical activities, and good health care, heart disease is avoidable. And if it is not avoided, it is treatable and certainly not a death sentence.

In cardiology, Metabolic Syndrome is known as the lethal quartet. True as that may be, it can be countered with positive steps. This chapter has concentrated on the "negatives" of heart disease. We have had to look at the "bad" things that we do to ourselves that can lead to cardiovascular problems and disease–the lethal quartet. Throughout the remainder of the book we will be delving into what I call the quartet for life, the four positive steps you can take to avoid heart Metabolic Syndrome and heart disease: Proper diet, adequate movement, low-stress environment, and benevolent attitude toward life. Continue with me on this journey to learn what you can do to ensure a long, healthy life free from cardiac disease.

Ease Your Way into Exercise
If you are going to take up a new exercise regimen, take these steps first:
- Have your family physician perform a complete physical. Tell him or her of your plans and get their feedback on your approach.
- Buy a quality pair of shoes. Select shoes designed for the type of exercise you will be doing. It is worth your money to go to a well-respected running store or shoe store in order to be fit by a professional. Shoes go a long way in reducing the risk of an injury, particularly for runners and walkers.
- Ease your way into exercise. Start with just a few minutes a day, 3 times a week, and gradually increase the duration and effort. In the running world, the common rule of thumb is to increase the duration of exercise by less than 10% a week.
- Keep your breathing even. You should be able to hold a conversation while exercising. If you are breathing so hard that this is not possible, you are exerting yourself too much. The goal is to keep your heart rate at a reasonable elevated level but not to elevate it into the "aerobic" range.

HEALTHY STEPS

- ♥ Proper diet
- ♥ Adequate activity
- ♥ Limited stressors
- ♥ Positive perspective

CHAPTER 4

Heart Disease in Women

Disease Is a Process

When a disease is diagnosed, it can feel like lightning has struck. If the diagnosis is cancer, the news can be devastating. After all, the patient likely felt fine with just a few niggling concerns. Their doctor may have told them, initially, that the blood tests were just a precaution, nothing serious. When the true illness is revealed, everything changes for that person. I have often been thankful that I did not practice the type of medicine where I would have to present that type of news.

For the person being diagnosed, it must seem as if the disease came out of nowhere. One day fine, the next day, wham! It can be a similar feeling when a heart attack occurs. All too often, the person has no indication of what their future holds. However, disease does not strike "out of the blue." It is a process that gradually reveals itself in subtle ways. If the subtleties are not diagnosed, eventually the disease will present itself in a major way, leaving no doubt as to the patient's condition.

Take for example any of the various forms of cancer. They all start at a basic genetic level, where one tiny gene mutates, throwing the entire biological process off. Sometimes the cancer will grow a tumor, as in breast or ovarian cancer. Sometimes it will wreak havoc in the bone marrow and create abnormal blood cells, as in leukemia. Whatever the case, the disease runs a fairly defined course. Unfortunately, in the case of most cancers, the causes are still ill-defined and much research has yet to be done. In the case of heart disease, we have some very clear preventative measures that, if undertaken, can short-circuit the disease process.

As you are reading through this chapter, I want you to keep in mind the risk factors we discussed earlier. Look at each heart condition that we are about to discuss as a process that started years before the diagnosis. In some cases, the

---

True Medical Story

A man came into the ER yelling, "My wife's going to have her baby in the cab!" The ER physician grabbed his stuff, rushed out to the cab, lifted the lady's dress, and just finished yanking off her underwear when he suddenly discovered that there were several cabs lined up, and it was obvious that he was in the wrong one.

---

process may have started in childhood. In many ways, if one has a genetic predisposition, the process will have begun before birth. Try to follow each one, from its opening stages to the end stages, and look for ways, at each stage, to circumvent the progression of the disease. That is what health is all about: mitigating risks and being proactive in caring for the body.

Atherosclerotic Disease

By far, the most common contributor to heart disease in women is atherosclerosis, also known as "hardening of the arteries." It is a natural process of aging, but the process can be accelerated by poor diet, stress, smoking, and many of the other risk factors we have already discussed. In order to better understand this disease process, you need to understand the circulatory system as a whole, from the formation of blood to the pumping action of the heart.

Of course, understanding the circulatory system in women is not as simple as comprehending the science. Over millennia, the image of blood has taken on complicated overtones. It means so much more to our imagination than science can explain. Blood has been symbolized in contradictory terms: it contaminates and purifies, convicts and redeems, gives and takes life. If you love vampire novels, blood may have an erotic overtone. For women, blood symbolizes menstruation, a central piece of the feminine nature.

Too Much of a Good Thing

Raynaud's phenomenon mimics atherosclerosis in some ways. It is a condition that causes the vessels in the fingers, toes, nose, and/or ears to spasm when they are exposed to cold or emotional stress. Typically, the affected area turns white, then blue, then bright red over the course of the attack. There may be associated tingling, swelling, or painful throbbing. The attacks may last from minutes to hours. In severe cases, the area may develop ulcerations and infections, which can lead to gangrene.

Women are nine times more likely than men to have Raynaud's. It is estimated to be present in 20% of women in their childbearing years. It can occur by itself or in the presence of an autoimmune disease, such as lupus.

The best treatment is to avoid cold temperature. Biofeedback has been effective in minimizing symptoms, particularly when they are aggravated by stress. If biofeedback is unsuccessful, drugs that dilate the vessels may provide some relief.

The "primitive" imagination searched for mystical explanations when it could not explain things physically. Blood was the most visible presence of the mysterious inner nature of the human body. It was obvious that blood brought death on the battlefield—warriors bathed in it. In contrast, many cultures believed babies were formed from the absent menstrual blood that congealed within a woman's womb. In this case, it was obviously responsible for life.

In current times, we can explain many things in physical terms, but the circulatory system, the most powerful force in human physiology, still contains many mysteries. It is an intricate feat of transportation engineering. It would be impossible to replicate anything like it with the technology we have today. For example, there are 100,000 miles of blood vessels in the adult body; laid out from end to end—that is enough to circle the earth four times. The circulatory system contains arteries as large as a straw and capillaries so small that only one blood cell can pass through at a time.

The circulatory system is responsible for carrying oxygen, nutrients, and other substances throughout the body and removing carbon dioxide and waste that is created during metabolism, digestion, and other processes. Without it, we would suffocate and starve; we would fall prey to sickness caused by our own wastes. So, in a sense, the ancients' beliefs are correct. The circulatory system is responsible for life, death, strength, and cleansing. Let's take a look at where it all starts.

The Life of a Blood Cell

Healthy blood is necessary for a functioning circulatory system, and it leads a rather miraculous existence. It is formed in the marrow of our bones, with the largest percentage created in the larger bones such as the hip, sternum, and thigh. Blood cells start as undifferentiated stem cells, meaning these "baby" cells have the potential to become any of the three major types of mature blood cells: whites, reds, and platelets. Complicated chemical reactions will determine what form a stem cell will take.

Red blood cells are the simplest of the three. They are basically empty blobs whose only job is to carry oxygen to the tissues of the body. Hemoglobin is the substance within the cell that attracts and carries the oxygen. Our lungs may be working perfectly, but without red blood cells, we would suffocate.

Table 4.1
Types of Blood Cells

Type of Cell	Function
Platelets (Thrombocytes)	Repair of vessels, clot formation
Red Blood Cells (Erythrocytes)	Transport of oxygen and carbon dioxide
White Blood Cells (Leukocytes)	Fight infections, combat allergens
subtypes of white blood cells	
Neutrophils	Main defense against bacteria
Eosinophils	Kill parasites, play a role in allergic reactions
Basophils	Function in allergic reactions
Monocytes	Kill bacteria, "clean up" old and dead cells
Lymphocytes	Direct the immune system

Women typically carry slightly less hemoglobin than men and consequently have a lower oxygen-carrying capacity. This means the most to elite endurance athletes, such as marathoners, who need every bit of oxygen they can get. Even so, there are over 5,000,000 red blood cells in a SINGLE drop of blood.

Oxygenated red blood cells (RBC) are what give blood its red color. Blood that is returning from the lungs is typically a bluish color. You can see the difference if you look at the arteries and veins on your arms. RBCs have a relatively long life and may live as long as 120 days.

White blood cells are warriors. Their job is to seek out and fight infection. Some of them, like granulocytes, "roll" along the walls of the veins searching for bacteria to eat. Others, like the monocytes migrate into the tissue and remove debris and other dangerous invaders. White blood cells have various life spans, living from days to weeks.

One of the great mysteries of these "infection-fighting" cells appears in newborns. Anecdotally, we know that baby boys have more difficulty fighting infections than do baby girls. We have yet to explain this scientifically, but talk to any neonatal nurse and they will tell you their preemie baby boys seem to be more fragile and susceptible to infection then baby girls.

Platelets are the final type of blood cell. They are irregularly shaped and mesh together to form clots at sites that are bleeding. Without platelets, as in the case of hemophilia, even a small bump can be a devastating injury because the body has no way of "sealing off" the wound.

All of these blood cells live within a fluid called the plasma, which is 90% water. Its usefulness may seem unremarkable compared to that of the blood cells, but plasma is like a river, and the cells are like fish. Without plasma, the cells would be without a stream. This pale yellow fluid also carries proteins, electrolytes (such as sodium and chloride), sugars, fats, waste products, amino acids, hormones, and vitamins. It is continually being cleansed by the liver and kidneys.

Obviously, this life-sustaining blood needs a system capable of carrying it throughout the body. We call that structure the cardiovascular system.

The Cardiovascular System

This contains blood and distributes it to the tissues. Arteries, veins, and capillaries are the three main structures.

Arteries take blood away from the heart. The blood in our arteries is carrying oxygen and nutrients. Veins carry blood back to the heart. They return blood that needs to be oxygenated so it can continue on to the body. Capillaries are the smallest of these structures. There are so small that there is one capillary near each CELL in your body. At their endpoint, the capillary walls exchange nutrients, wastes, and gases.

The "S"-Word Again
Heavy exertion and overeating are more likely to trigger a heart attack in men, whereas mental stress was more commonly associated with the onset in women.

You can think of the circulatory system as a figure-eight. Blood starts in the left ventricle of the aorta (the lower-left corner of the heart) and circulates to the body, depositing oxygen and nutrients along the way. It returns through venules, veins, and the vena cava to the right ventricle of the heart. From here, the pulmonary artery carries it to the lungs, where alveoli (tiny air sacs in the lungs) exchange carbon dioxide for oxygen. The oxygenated blood goes back to the heart through the pulmonary vein into the left atrium (the upper-left corner of the heart) and finally the left ventricle, where the entire process repeats.

The coronary arteries supply the heart with oxygenated blood. They can provide seven ounces a minute to the surface of the heart. That is 4-5% of the total blood volume, even though the heart is less than 1% of the total body weight. Any muscle in the body needs oxygen to continue to flex and relax; however, the heart muscle must do this over three billion times in your life. It requires huge amounts of oxygen, and hence a large blood supply, to function.

This technical discussion about the circulatory system was designed to give you the background to understand the process of atherosclerosis—why it can be devastating and how it can be prevented. Atherosclerosis is actually a disease that manifests itself in many ways: coronary artery disease, stroke, peripheral-vascular disease, renal-artery stenosis, carotid-artery stenosis, and cerebrovascular disease. We will concern ourselves primarily with the first three, since they are the most closely related to your cardiac function. However, before we go on to discuss them, let's look in on Sarah.

Sarah's Story

I heard the words "estrogen…menopause…starts with nicks in the blood vessels." I was listening to the doctor, but his words were making little sense to me. Earlier in the evening, I gratefully crawled into bed for some much-needed rest, and the next thing I know my husband is calling an ambulance because I've become so sick that I am lapsing in and out of consciousness. I don't remember much from the time I hit the bed to the time I woke up in the hospital except for an incredible pain in my chest and a lot of doctors and nurses all around me—those images, and the words "Sarah, you are having a heart attack. Hang in there. We are doing our best to help you." How could I have known that I would ever hear those words in my life, let alone on this particular night?

"Sarah, do you have any questions?" The doctor was hurried, ready to move on to the next set of complications, but I was still trying to make the emotional pieces fit. I had lost my father to a heart attack nearly five years earlier and the ugly beast was in my life again. I was holding my mother's hand. Where once there had been thick, supple skin there was now a papery sheath covering a network of vessels. Her outer wrapping may be thin, but her heart and strength are not. I'm glad she is here with me to make sense of all this.

The doctor patiently explained that coronary disease is caused by the hardening of the arteries, the big word being atherosclerosis. He said it was a byproduct of age, smoking, and other incremental insults. Normally, the lining of our veins is slippery and smooth, allowing blood to flow smoothly. When the lining gets scratched, it allows cholesterol in the blood to take hold and form a streak that becomes layered with more plaque, until eventually the vessel is totally blocked.

Apparently smoking is one of the things that cause damage to this sensitive lining. As a young girl, I watched my mother's every move—my small fingers would imitate the "cigarette pose" as my lips pursed into a bow to blow smoke rings. Smoking was a rite of passage for me. I would sneak off with my girlfriends during lunch break at school. We had to hide from the teachers, but had to be seen by the other kids or the drama of it all was lost. I smoked in defiance of my parents but in harmony with their own example.

To make matters worse, diet was a four-letter word in our house. My parents had lived through the Depression, and they made up for every moment of it by preparing huge meals and expecting us to "eat up or waste away." My mother was a wonderful cook and my father followed close behind. They took turns preparing the big family meal on Sunday, a tradition we still keep even though Dad is gone.

The doctor was still looking at me, waiting for a question or response of some kind. I'd asked my questions. I didn't know where to go next.

I examined my mother's face to get a hint of what must be going on in her mind. Her expression was noncommittal, and I assumed she was weighing all the options.

"Sarah, would you like to discuss the surgery?" the doctor was again, trying to make sure he had our attention. It must be obvious that my focus was divided between the present and the past.

"Go ahead, Doctor." My mother spoke for me. Her voice was worn and soft.

"I am proposing a coronary-artery-bypass graft. We use the acronym cabbage (CABG) for short. We will take a vein from the leg and graft it to the artery that is blocked. This will effectively route the blood flow around the portion of the artery that is blocked. Over 300,000 of these surgeries are done in the United States every year, and there is every reason to believe that you will tolerate the procedure well. However, we do know women have a more difficult time in recovery than men do. You will need at least six weeks before you will be feeling somewhat normal again."

He searched his hands as he spoke as if they contained the words he needed to clearly explain such an obviously complicated surgery.

"I understand the basics of the surgery, Doctor. I still don't understand how we didn't catch this sooner. Why didn't we know about this problem before it came to this?" My mother's tone bordered on confrontational. She was clearly concerned.

"Well, we know the most common sign of heart disease in men is chest pain. However, less than 70% of women with coronary artery disease complain of it, and when they do, it is usually after months or years of suffering with it. By that time, they may have other problems that mask the symptoms, such as osteoporosis or arthritis. Your headache and nausea, along with complaints of fatigue, were indicators, but most people don't know that until it is too late."

I turned to my mother. "Mom, do you understand all of this?"

"Not completely, but I trust the doctor." Her eyes were darker than normal. No sign of her trademark sparkle.

"I know you must both be scared, but a successful surgery will have you feeling better than you have felt in months. We could consider managing the condition with medications and diet, but at this point the disease is advanced enough that we need to address the blockage. I believe this is the best option for you at this time."

The doctor took my hand as he stood up. "Please let me know if you have any other concerns; otherwise, we will see you in surgery tomorrow."

"That soon, Doctor?" The knot in my stomach told me I definitely was not pre-pared. I squeezed my mother's hand. I hadn't told my children or talked to my husband. They were waiting at home for me, expecting to see me walk through the door at any moment, but at the age of forty-five, I was facing surgery or certain

death. My children would be without a mother and my husband without a wife. There was a chance I would succumb to the same fate as my father.

"I need to talk to my family."

"Of course. They will cope better if they know the full truth. Let them support you, but talk to them tonight."

He turned toward the door, his back bent just a bit. "I'll see you in the morning. Thanks, ladies." And with that he was gone, on to the next patient, the next heart, the next set of problems to be solved.

Coronary Artery Disease (CAD)

Coronary artery disease—we'll use CAD for short—has long been thought to be a man's disease, but we now know that nothing could be further from the truth. Women are dying in alarming numbers, well over 250,000 every year. It is clear that the medical world needs to get a handle on this disease process in women. The first step is to educate women so that they might reduce their risks and increase their chances of avoiding a potentially devastating illness. Equally as important, women must receive the same research attention as men do. It was not until the early 1980s that science began to view women as equally at risk for heart disease. It is not until very recently that science began to view women as being wholly different from men with respect to heart disease. We are now finding that the physiologic differences have a major impact on how heart disease presents itself and that women have unique risks for acquiring it. I'd like to present some of these specific differences and give you a brief overview of CAD and how it might affect you.

Definitions

Coronary artery disease: disease caused by blocked arteries

Coronary heart disease: damage to heart muscle from coronary artery disease

Cardiovascular disease: any disease that affects the heart or the blood vessels

The coronary arteries supply blood directly to the heart. They overlie the heart in a "crown-like" fashion and are directly responsible for feeding the muscle tissue of the heart.

Studies have shown women have smaller coronary arteries (Sheifer 2000). This makes sense in that women are typically smaller than men. However, even when the researchers adjusted for size, it appeared that these are arteries are smaller in women.

Did You Know?
You heart will have pumped an average of 48 million gallons by the time you are 70.

For years, it was believed that women had a worse outcome than men with respect to heart disease because of their smaller stature. However, this study has proven that regardless of size, women's arteries are smaller. There is a sex-specific influence acting on arterial size. This smaller size allows the arteries to clog more readily. They are also more difficult to operate on.

As for the implications of the study, Dr. Sheifer writes, "If specific mechanisms for sex differences are identified, they could ultimately serve as targets for novel therapies aimed at increasing coronary size. Given that prior studies have suggested that coronary artery size has prognostic implications, such therapies hold the potential to improve outcomes of women with coronary artery disease." We hope it is not long before scientists identify these compounds and are able to use them to increase the size of women's arteries and improve the outcome of their heart disease.

Typically, the interior of the veins and arteries is very smooth and blood flows freely. With age, the arteries lose their elasticity and become more brittle due to calcium content. This is a natural process of aging called atherosclerosis, and it varies in seriousness in each individual.

Another side effect of aging is the buildup of fatty deposits. The originally smooth lining of the arteries becomes damaged over time and begins to collect "fatty streaks," often as early as the teen years. Eventually, these streaks collect more fats and plaque. After a time, this plaque can build up and affect circulation and blood pressure. It can progress to the point of completely blocking the blood flow in a coronary artery. This can result in sudden death from a heart attack.

Atherosclerosis can occur anywhere in the body, but it is particularly troublesome when it happens in the coronary arteries. These arteries are completely responsible for supplying the heart with the oxygen it needs. When the heart muscle is deprived of oxygen for any length of time, it begins to die. This typically results in a heart attack, and you may or may not be aware of it.

Women's arteries are protected by the natural production of estrogen prior to menopause. It helps to keep your vessels flexible. It protects the inner lining of your arteries, as well. This is important, because it is the small nicks in the inner lining of the blood vessel that allow plaque to adhere to the vessel and begin to build up. Estrogen also decreases the level of blood sugar, which is the primary culprit in damaging the sensitive inner lining of the vessels.

Estrogen is responsible for stimulating the production of a factor (endothelial cell-releasing factor) that stimulates the vessels to dilate, which leads to blood flowing more easily. If a vessel is clogged it may not dilate normally. We know that estrogen encourages the release of this factor in the coronary arteries of post-menopausal women with atherosclerosis.

There are many other triggers that can cause the arteries to contract, including stress. If your vessels are already narrowed from plaque build-up, any additional contraction can be harmful.

On the extreme of CAD is a heart attack, though it can happen that the first symptom of CAD is a heart attack. Even worse, a heart attack can be "silent," meaning there were no obvious symptoms that it was occurring. This can be brought on by the simple narrowing of the arteries or by a blood clot forming in the vessel. When plaque builds up on the lining of a vessel, it has a hard outer shell and a center of soft cholesterol. If the hard shell cracks, a blood clot will form at the site. This may completely block the flow of blood in that vessel, leading to a heart attack.

What to Look For

Women tend to develop CAD about ten years later, on average, than men. This is thought to be related to the production of estrogen.

What to Expect During an Electrocardiogram

EKGs are quick, safe, and painless. You will be instructed to lie down. A technician will clean a total of ten areas on your chest and apply a special conductive gel, similar to the gel used during an ultrasound. Then the tech will apply ten small pads (electrodes) to each of these areas. These electrodes are connected to the EKG machine. You will be asked to lie as still as possible for about a minute or so while the electrodes record your heart activity. Each electrode creates a "tracing" on a strip of paper. These tracings, when compared against each other, paint a unique picture of the activity of your heart. Your doctor can read them and interpret a variety of conditions from the patterns seen there.

You may be asked to walk on a treadmill at different speeds and elevations to measure your heart during exercise, as well.

Once women pass fifty, they surpass men in the incidence and mortality due to CAD. Over 350,000 women die each year from CAD.

Common risk factors for CAD include cigarette smoking, high cholesterol, high blood pressure, diabetes, family history, and obesity.

Because the majority of studies have been done with men as the primary subjects, the "typical" symptom seen is angina. This is described as a chest discomfort that is brought on by exertion and relieved by rest or taking nitroglycerin. However, while this may predict CAD in men 93% of the time, it only works for women 72% of the time.

There may be several reasons for this. One is that by the time women develop CAD, they have also developed other diseases that can make it difficult to diagnose. Arthritis and osteoporosis are two such conditions. Also, women do not report chest pain as often as they report abdominal pain, difficulty breathing, nausea, or fatigue. Often women delay seeking treatment for these symptoms. They may suffer for years before bringing it to the attention of their doctor. Unfortunately, chest pain in women is also often chalked up to anxiety, stress, and other psychological problems.

Testing

The traditional means of testing for CAD has been exercise electrocardiography. This is the typical treadmill test that you may have seen on TV or represented elsewhere in the media. It is not necessarily the best test for women, as the results can be skewed by hormonal interactions and physical characteristics. Exercise echocardiography is a better choice. This test is an ultrasound performed before and after exercise. It is noninvasive and has been shown to have the best sensitivity in determining the presence of CAD in women. MRI and CAT scans are also coming onto the scene as promising new ways to test for heart disease and heart attack.

Treatment

Women need to pay particular attention to the diagnosis of CAD. Studies have shown that men are ten times more likely to be referred for further testing if they have an abnormal stress test (Tobin 1987). It is essential that you insist on further testing if you have unexplained chest pain or an abnormal stress test. If it is determined that you have CAD, there are several treatments available. However, a coronary-artery-bypass graft (CABG) and balloon dilation (also known as angioplasty) are the most common interventions. These procedures carry special risks for women and should not be undertaken lightly. Your best offense is a good defense. Reduce your risk factors wherever possible and follow the recommendations we outline in this book for decreasing your susceptibility.

Angioplasty

Angioplasty is used to re-open arteries that have been blocked by plaque buildup. The doctor will use a local anesthetic to numb the upper thigh area above the femoral artery. A very thin tube with a tiny balloon is inserted into the artery. The physician watches the balloon advance through the artery until it reaches the site of the blockage. The balloon is then inflated, pushing the plaque back against the wall of the artery. The balloon is then withdrawn and often a stent (wire-mesh tube) is left behind. The stent keeps the artery open and allows blood to flow freely.

Most importantly, pay attention to your body and the signals it sends you. Women have different means of processing physical pain than men and often "write off" chest pain and other indicators. Your heart will communicate. You must be willing to listen to it and treat it with the seriousness it deserves. Trust your intuition and don't let your healthcare providers convince you it is "all in your mind" or "just anxiety." If you feel it is physically based, odds are you are correct. The worst outcome is that you would be submitted to a test that turns up negative. That is a far better outcome than a heart attack down the line.

CORONARY ARTERY DIESEASE (CAD)—SUMMARY

Risk Factors
- ♥ Diabetes
- ♥ Smoking
- ♥ Sedentary lifestyle
- ♥ Postmenopausal age
- ♥ Family History
- ♥ Stress

Symptoms in Women
- ♥ Shoulder, jaw, or neck pain
- ♥ Nausea
- ♥ Fatigue
- ♥ Shortness of breath

Testing
- ♥ Exercise-tolerance test
- ♥ Exercise echocardiogram
- ♥ Variety of other imaging studies
- ♥ Cardiac catheterization

Treatment
- ♥ Cholesterol-lowering drugs
- ♥ Angioplasty
- ♥ Bypass surgery

Prognosis
- ♥ Women are more likely to die of a first heart attack
- ♥ Women experience more long-term disability
- ♥ Women have high incidence of other illnesses

Prevention
- ♥ Proper diet and exercise
- ♥ Smoking cessation
- ♥ Cholesterol-lowering drugs
- ♥ Reduction of "bad" stress

Stroke

Can you imagine having awareness of your environment but not being able to express yourself either verbally or physically? How difficult would it be to listen to your loved ones talk without being able to respond appropriately? A stroke can have a devastating impact physically and emotionally. Their effects are unpredictable. Some women may suffer very slight symptoms that last for just a few minutes while other strokes can leave a person in a vegetative state. Unfortunately, strokes take the lives of over 100,000 women every year. Clearly this is a health threat that women need to take seriously. There is no cure for a stroke once it has happened, but there are many avenues to prevention.

There are three types of stroke that are closely related to cardiovascular disease, and because strokes and heart attacks are both caused by blood clots, the treatment is

---

What Is a Septal Defect?

A septal defect occurs when the closure between the two upper chambers of the heart is not tight. This allows blood to flow through the hole or defect from one chamber to the other, causing the other chambers to pump extra blood.

---

surprisingly similar. A cerebral embolism is caused by small pieces of cholesterol sloughing off the lining of the arteries in the neck and traveling until they reach a smaller branch in the vessel and become wedged. This blocks further blood flow. A cerebral thrombosis is caused by atherosclerosis or a blood clot that forms and stays in the artery in the neck or brain in which it is formed. It does not move from the spot it is formed in, but it does inhibit blood flow.

Rarely, a stroke can be caused by a blood clot that forms in a leg vein, breaks away, and crosses through to the left side of the heart by way of a septal defect and then proceeds into an artery of the brain. Often this may be the first indication of a septal defect. There are other types of strokes that can be the first sign of heart disease, including a stroke caused by a blood clot formed at an aging valve.

What to Look For

The risk factors for stroke are very similar to those for hardening of the arteries. They include high blood pressure, smoking, physical inactivity, high cholesterol, and obesity. This is another case for establishing healthy habits as early as possible in life, although it is never too late. If you have these risk factors, it is important to mitigate them in the best way you possibly can.

The "traditional" symptoms of stroke are sudden changes in—
- ♥ Sensation
- ♥ Walking ability
- ♥ Motor function

♥ Speech
♥ Use of language
♥ Facial muscles
♥ Vision
♥ Balance (or dizziness)

These are the traditional symptoms because they are commonly seen in males having a stroke. However, recent studies have shown, not surprisingly, that women often have very different symptoms. The danger here is that, as with a heart attack, a stroke needs to be treated immediately. The same anti-clotting agents used in a heart attack will often be used to treat a stroke. The sooner they are given, the less damage will be caused to the brain.

Overall, 28% of women versus 19% of men report "nontraditional" symptoms, such as—

♥ Headache
♥ Face pain
♥ Limb pain
♥ Disorientation and change in consciousness
♥ Hiccups
♥ Nausea
♥ General Weakness
♥ Chest pain
♥ Shortness of breath
♥ Palpitations

Women's symptoms are less specific, which could lead to further delay in detecting the stroke. (Labiche et al. 2002)

Treatment

The only cure for a stroke is prevention. If you have any of the risk factors mentioned, it is important to work with them and do your best to reduce them. Once a stroke happens, only fate will determine how your brain will be affected. After a mini-stroke, the damage may last less than a day. A major stroke can cause death. In fact, women fare worse then men after a stroke, so it is even more important for you to consider ways to reduce your risk. The good news is that the same steps to a healthy heart will lead you to stroke prevention.

There are studies being conducted with respect to "estrogen-specific" drugs that are used to treat osteoporosis. Preliminary findings show that they cut the risks of non-fatal strokes by 68%, but more conclusive findings aren't due out until 2005.

There are also indications that in the fourth and fifth decade of life, blood flow in the arteries is greatly reduced in women as compared to men. This means that other vessels are not able to compensate as well for a blockage or reduction in blood flow in blocked vessels. This sets the stage for a potential stroke.

All of us, especially women, need to examine the way we deal with the stress in our lives. It has been shown that women who experience a rise in blood pressure and heart rate during mental stress may develop accelerated athero-sclerosis. Women who respond with a pulse pressure increase also have thicker vessel linings and more plaque, precursors to heart attack and stroke. Stress also releases chemicals into the bloodstream that negatively stimulate the heart muscle and increase blood pressure.

If you demonstrate any signs of a stroke or have any suspicion that you may have had a mini-stroke, it is vital to get medical care immediately.

STROKE—SUMMARY

Risk Factors
- ♥ Diabetes
- ♥ High blood pressure
- ♥ Smoking
- ♥ Obesity
- ♥ High cholesterol
- ♥ Physical inactivity
- ♥ Stress

Symptoms in Women
- ♥ Pain or headache
- ♥ Changes in consciousness or disorientation
- ♥ Chest pain
- ♥ Shortness of breath
- ♥ Difficulty speaking
- ♥ Facial drooping, particularly on one side
- ♥ Clumsiness or inability to walk
- ♥ Weakness or numbness on one side of the body
- ♥ Dizziness/vertigo
- ♥ Changes in sensation
- ♥ Visual problems

Testing
- ♥ Usually based on neurological assessment
- ♥ Carotid Doppler
- ♥ Three-dimensional carotid MRA

Treatment
- ♥ Cholesterol-lowering drugs
- ♥ Carotid endarterectomy

Prognosis
- ♥ Women are more likely than men to die or have a poor outcome after a stroke.
- ♥ More women than men die of stroke.
- ♥ Women who have a stroke face longer delays than men in being evaluated by emergency-room physicians, leading to a worse outcome.

Prevention
- ♥ Proper diet and exercise
- ♥ Blood pressure-lowering drugs
- ♥ Smoking cessation
- ♥ Cholesterol-lowering drugs
- ♥ Reduction of "bad" stress

Peripheral Vascular Disease

There was a popular song a few years ago with the words, "I would walk 500 miles/And I would walk 500 more/Just to be the man who walked 1000 miles to fall down at your door." At the time, I thought this was a very romantic depiction of a human's tenacity and resilience when it comes to love. I also reflected on the nature of walking and what it means to us. In this age of automobiles and public transit, we don't often call on our innate ability to transport ourselves by walking. We take for granted something that we struggled with almost exclusively for the first few years of our life. Once mastered, the skill becomes a much taken-for-granted ability that we appreciate too little—at least, until it fails us.

Peripheral vascular disease (PVD) is one of the health issues that can cause us to lose our ability to walk, or at least to walk any distance free from pain.

PVD is caused by atherosclerosis in the "periphery" of the body, namely the arms and legs. It is most common in the legs but can occur anywhere. If you have PVD, it may be an indicator of atherosclerosis in your coronary arteries and/or your brain. If you are diagnosed with PVD, it is important that your doctor check you for signs and symptoms of these disease processes as well.

Are You at Risk for Peripheral Vascular Disease?
Take this quick quiz to assess your risk for PVD.
1. Do you smoke?
2. Do others in your household smoke?
3. Do you exercise less than three times a week?
4. Are you overweight?
5. Is your cholesterol intake lower than acceptable American Heart Association guidelines?
6. Does your fat intake exceed the American Heart Association guidelines?
7. Do you eat fewer than five servings of vegetables and/or fruits a day?
8. Are you over 45?
9. Do you have coronary artery disease?
If you answer "yes" to four or more of these questions, you are considered to be "at risk" for peripheral vascular disease. Be sure to have a screening and follow-up performed by your physician.
Courtesy of Guidant at *www.guidant.com*

The risk factors for PVD are the same as for other forms of atherosclerosis, which we have already discussed. Smoking is a greater risk for PVD than for the other forms by a great degree. It is also greatly complicated by diabetes, which increases the risk of intermittent claudication (pain in the legs caused by lack of oxygen to the muscles) by three times. This is a particularly dangerous condition for diabetics, because they often develop ulcers in the skin tissue that are difficult to heal.

What to Look For

The primary symptoms of PVD are pain, aching, fatigue, or discomfort in the lower extremities while walking that goes away when one stops. Pain in the foot at rest (ischemic rest pain) is another symptom. If you have any of these symptoms or other signs of atherosclerosis, such as mini-strokes, chest discomfort, or previous heart attack, you should ask your doctor to check you out for PVD. Over 60% of patients with PVD also have CAD, and about 40% of patients with PVD also have a history of stroke.

As PVD worsens, the symptoms may progress to numbness and tingling in the toes, foot, and leg; paleness of the foot or leg when elevated; a blue or red discoloration when the leg is hanging; absence of pulse in the foot; coldness in the foot and leg; or a sore on the foot that does not heal.

You Diagnose It

Sophie was only 18 years old when she was first referred to my office. She had been experiencing palpitations and feelings of lightheadedness. Her mother told me that she had always been a healthy child, with no serious illnesses. Sophie assured me that she was not using any drugs.

Upon examination, I found her pulse to be about 270 beats per minute and regular. Her blood pressure was 100/60. She was having a bit of difficulty breathing normally. Her EKG showed an abnormal wave pattern.

Discussion

Because Sophie assured me she was not using drugs, I ruled out cocaine use or other drug-related causes for her rapid heart rate. Her EKG told the true story. Sophie had a syndrome called Wolfe-Parkinson-White. The actual incidence of WPW Syndrome is not known, but most reports say that it appears in 0.1 to 3 per 1000 EKGs.

WPW Syndrome is a defect in the conduction of the electrical impulses of the heart. There is an "extra" connection between the upper chambers and the lower chambers, causing the rapid heart rate. In very rare cases, it can be a cause of sudden death, but most often it goes undetected.

In Sophie's case, it was causing her difficulty, so we decided to treat it with radiofrequency ablation. This would take away the need for long-term medication and most likely provide a long-lasting cure.

Radiofrequency ablation is done by threading a wire into the heart through the femoral artery. The abnormal pathway is located by electrical stimulation and destroyed by passing a high current through it. The treatment takes 2-3 hours and usually requires a night in the hospital.

In Sophie's case, it corrected the rhythm problems entirely. She follows up with me once every couple of years to have an EKG, but otherwise lives her life normally, with no untoward side effects.

Testing

There are several tests your doctor can perform to detect PVD. The first and most common is called the ankle/brachial index. This number is arrived at by using a Doppler ultrasound to record the systolic blood pressures in your arms and legs. This test is highly sensitive and a strong indicator of the severity and prognosis of the disease. There are other tests that can be done in a vascular laboratory. Your doctor may choose to use them if he or she needs more detail on the severity and location of the disease.

If you have PVD, it is important that your doctor check for other types of atherosclerosis, such as CAD. It is likely that you will demonstrate this condition in other arteries in your body.

Treatment

The standard treatment for PVD is daily aspirin. There are also some other drugs, called antiplatelet drugs, that can prevent your blood from forming clots that lead to stroke. They are very effective and well-tested. There are a few other drugs, such as ramipril, Cilostazol, and pentoxifylline, that have been used with success as well. L-arginine is a drug that is currently under study and shows some potential in helping women suffering with PVD.

Exercise is the best form of treatment for PVD. A study published January 2003 (McDermott) demonstrated that women suffering from PVD have more difficulty walking than men that are suffering from the same disease. Part of the explanation is that men have more leg strength than women. However, they also found that men tend to walk more in their leisure time, whereas women got a significant amount of their physical activity from housework. Exercise can trigger leg pain, so it is difficult to walk regularly, but it will help over the long-term by prolonging the amount of time you can walk pain-free. It is also shown that regular exercise may prevent elderly people with PVD from requiring nursing home care. Get out and walk, walk, walk.

PERIPHERAL VASCULAR DISEASE (PVD)—SUMMARY

Risk Factors
- ♥ Advanced age
- ♥ Cigarette smoking
- ♥ Diabetes
- ♥ High blood pressure
- ♥ High cholesterol
- ♥ Excessive alcohol consumption
- ♥ Hyperhomocysteinemia

Symptoms in Women
- ♥ Pain, aching, fatigue, or discomfort in the lower extremities while walking which stops when walking stops
- ♥ Numbness and tingling in the toe, foot and leg
- ♥ Paleness of the foot or leg when elevated
- ♥ Blue or red discoloration when the leg is hanging
- ♥ Absence of pulse in the foot
- ♥ Coldness in the foot and leg
- ♥ A sore on the foot that doesn't heal

Testing
- ♥ Ankle/brachial index
- ♥ Duplex ultrasonography
- ♥ Segmental limb pressures
- ♥ Vascular examination, including listening for and feeling for pulse in the upper and lower extremity arteries, abdomen, and neck; complete blood count; blood-cholesterol level testing; blood-sugar level testing; and urinalysis.

Treatment
- ♥ Reduce risk factors: stop smoking, lower blood pressure, lower cholesterol, and exercise.
- ♥ Antiplatelet therapy (heparin)
- ♥ Ramipril (Altace)
- ♥ Cilostazol (Pletal)
- ♥ Pentoxifylline (Trental)

Prevention
- ♥ Proper diet and exercise
- ♥ Walk, walk, walk
- ♥ Smoking cessation
- ♥ Control blood sugars to avoid diabetes

Sarah's Story

One nice thing about hospitals is that there are no alarm clocks. The flip side is that it doesn't matter, because you don't get to sleep anyway. Unfamiliar sounds and smells, nurses in and out of the room, vital signs to check, medications to take, and the most uncomfortable beds in the world. I have been watching the clock tick off seconds for the last few hours. It's now 6:05, and the nurse should be here any minute to get me ready for the operating room. This has all happened so fast I still don't believe I'm here.

In the few minutes that I did manage to sleep last night, I dreamt about my children and my family. Josh was particularly upset when I explained to him that I was very sick and needed to have an operation. He was worried that he had made me sick by getting in the fight at school. He was worried that he could catch it. He was worried that he might never see me again. As a parent, how do you prepare yourself for the time when you have to face your young children, knowing that there is a possibility they might not see you alive again. How do you convince them of their innocence when they are so certain that they are the cause of the problem?

In the end, I did my best to reassure him, in spite of the tubes and machines clicking and swooshing all around us. We read a book together, just like we would do at home, and I sent him away with his dad to finish the nightly routine. If I can't be there for him, maybe the routine will provide him some comfort and security.

My mom is here to be with me while they get me ready. Her face is drawn, and my empathy for her is magnified. She is suffering as a mother for me just as I am for my own children. This common experience flows between us, and not a word needs to be spoken. I joke with her that she must have slept in the hospital too, as tired as she looks, and she fires back with a "mother-ism" about taking care of myself and forgetting about everyone else for awhile. She knows from experience that there is little chance of that. I am, after all, my mother's daughter.

Eventually, the nurse comes in once again to explain the surgery and get all of the appropriate consent forms signed. My mom takes in all the information and asks a few questions. I will actually be placed on a heart bypass machine that will circulate blood in place of my heart while the surgery is taking place. The doctor will "harvest" a vessel from my leg and use it to bypass the blocked vessels near my heart. The operating-room and staff are ready, and the nurse leaves to give my mom and me a few minutes to talk before they take me away.

She takes my hand and looks away, her tears pushing at the edges of her eyes. She sees it as her duty to stifle any feeling that might make me even slightly anx-

ious right now. Later I will worry about how to explain to her that it really causes me more anxiety to have her hide her emotions. Now, I just want to tell her thanks for being here now and thanks for being with me all the times I needed you. I want to reassure her that I will wake up on the other side of the surgery and that there will be many more moments for us. I want her to carry that hope to my husband and my children. I want her to carry it for me now, just for the next few hours.

Heart Failure

As a physician, I find the human heart to be a miracle of biology and spirit. My mother used to tell me there were two kinds of women. The first live to have powerful hearts full of love and grace. The second ease through life on tender threads, hoping to avoid the devastating grief of a broken heart. She wanted me to marry the first type but have compassion for the second.

"It is the women who have broken hearts that will be your patients," she told me one evening when after a long discussion about my future ambitions.

My mother meant it metaphorically, and though I was trained to treat women medically, I actually came to disagree with her on this point. I have worked with all types of women, most of them very loving and courageous. The physical strength of their hearts has little to do with their emotional strength, but our emotional lives do impact our hearts. This conversation with my mother raised an interesting question in my mind. Why are we so unwilling to accept that a woman's "physical" heart can be broken? Is it because we look at a man's broken heart as a necessary evil, something inevitable but fixable? Medicine has always shied away from the mysterious places that are not easily quantifiable. When a man has a broken heart he is expected to drink a few beers, slouch around for a few days, and get on with life. When a woman has a broken heart, the damage seems permanent and wholeness irretrievable.

Most women seem to have an innate ability to carry great pain and great joy at the same time. Men are often much more one-sided. Not that they don't experience their share of both, but they don't seem to mingle them. They are either in pain or in joy. Women are complicated in that they experience both simultaneously: the pain and joy of childbirth, the bittersweet emotions of sending their youngest off to kindergarten, the wedding of an only daughter.

Elizabeth Stone said having a child "is to decide forever to have your heart walk around outside your body." This keenly illuminates the central mystery of a woman's heart and why it is such a tricky thing to treat.

With all of that said, we are going to look at the medical context of a broken heart, a heart in failure. I want you to have a clear idea of how it presents in women and the best treatments we have available. If you happen to be one of the unfortunate 50% to be affected by heart disease, I want you to be an informed advocate for your care and understand the difference in the medical models used to treat men and women.

The Workhorse

The heart is an amazing piece of muscle. It contains its own electrical system that stimulates it to pump and an ingenious system of checks and balances to keep blood moving in the right direction in the right amounts. Furthermore, it must flex and contract billions of times over the course of one's life without getting tired!

The heart muscle squeezes together, creating a pumping action. It does this by coordinated contractions that shorten the muscle fibers. When the muscle relaxes, the fibers lengthen. Muscle contraction forces blood out and relaxation draws blood in. The heart has a sophisticated means of ensuring that equal amounts of blood go in and out. If the heart took in just a bit more blood than it pumped out, eventually the chambers would fill with blood and lose the ability to function.

When you have your blood pressure taken, you may hear the terms systole and diastole. Systole is the contraction phase of the heart. Diastole is the relaxation phase. The blood pressure cuff helps measure the pressure exerted against your veins when the heart is flexing (the systolic, or top, number) and relaxing (the diastolic, or bottom, number).

The heart doesn't work alone in its pumping mechanism. The leg muscles need to be moving to help propel blood toward the chest. If you are standing still, 15-20% of your blood pools in your legs. If this becomes exaggerated enough, it can cause you to feel dizzy or even pass out. Maybe this explains why so many grooms faint at the altar!

The heart pumps an average of one quart of blood per minute. Of that blood, 9% is traveling to and from your lungs, 7% is in your heart, and 85% is in the vessels traveling to tissues of your body. It takes a pretty powerful muscle to accomplish all this!

In spite of the miraculous ability of the heart, it can fail. Heart failure is a particularly devastating disease. It is actually many different diseases classified under one title. Although it suggests your heart has stopped entirely, that is not true. It is a process where the pumping action of the heart is no longer strong enough to supply the circulatory system with the pressure it needs to adequately circulate the blood. We will now look specifically at congestive heart failure and cardiomyopathy.

Drugs Used to Treat CHF

Positive Inotropic Medications: These drugs stimulate the contractions of the heart so that it is more efficient at pumping blood. Some of these drugs are digitalis, dopamine, dobutamine, and amrinone. Doctors don't like to use these drugs over long periods, because they may hasten the process of weakening the heart by forcing it to work too hard.

Vasodilators: It is possible to reduce the load the heart has to carry by dilating the vessels of the body. This results in less resistance to blood flow and allows the heart to work easier. The most popular form of these drugs are called ACE (angiotensin converting enzyme) inhibitors.

Diuretics: If you reduce the volume of blood by removing fluid accumulation, it will also make the work of the heart easier. These drugs are commonly used, and they are called diuretics. They promote urine production by the kidneys, which in turn reduces the amount of fluid retained by the body. They work quickly and vary in their potency.

Beta blockers: These drugs may slow the progression of the disease and improve symptoms by slowing the heart's contraction rate and reducing its pumping action. Increased adrenaline levels in the system are a sign of CHF. Beta blockers literally "block" the effects of adrenaline on the body.

Anticoagulants: Patients with heart failure are susceptible to blood clots within their heart or leg veins because their heart is not creating enough pumping pressure to effectively keep the blood moving. Warfarin is a common drug used to "thin" the blood and prevent coagulation.

Cardiotonics: These are intravenous drugs that increase the force of the heart's contractions.

Congestive Heart Failure

Congestive heart failure (CHF) is usually a symptom of cardiovascular disease as well as a disease process of its own. An equal number of men and women are diagnosed with heart failure every year. However, women die at a higher rate than men, about 45,000 deaths a year. There are different types of CHF. They are classified according to which side of the heart is more affected, which phase of the heartbeat is more affected, and how severe the condition is. Let's start with left versus right-sided CHF.

Left-sided CHF is characterized by the failure of the left ventricle to adequately pump blood from the heart to the rest of the body. The main symptom is shortness of breath. Fatigue, coughing, and lung congestion are other possible symptoms

Right-sided heart failure results in fluid build-up and edema, because the right ventricle is not applying enough pressure to keep blood circulating properly.

CHF can be classified according to the phase of the heart's pumping cycle that is more affected, systolic or diastolic.

Systolic failure means that the heart cannot pump enough blood during its contraction. Lung congestion is typically a result of this condition.

Diastolic failure happens when the heart cannot relax completely between contractions. Swelling in the abdomen and legs occurs frequently with this problem.

Finally, CHF can be evaluated based on its severity. This disease is usually progressive, and the New York Heart Association has identified four categories.

- ♥ Class I: No obvious symptoms, no limitations on physical activity
- ♥ Class II: Some symptoms during or after normal activity, mild physical activity limitations
- ♥ Class III: Symptoms with less-than-ordinary activity, moderate to significant physical activity limitations
- ♥ Class IV: Significant symptoms at rest, severe to total physical activity limitations

The American Heart Association estimates there are more than 5,000,000 people living with CHF. Studies have demonstrated that CHF most often occurs as a result of coronary artery disease, hypertension, and heart attacks.

Cardiomyopathy

Cardiomyopathy is a disease of the heart muscle that leads to heart failure. It is relatively uncommon but is the leading cause for heart transplant. There are three basic types of cardiomyopathy.

- ♥ **Dilated cardiomyopathy:** The heart muscle becomes weak and the chambers enlarge to compensate. This form often occurs in middle-aged people and more often in men than women.
- ♥ **Hypertrophic cardiomyopathy:** The heart muscle itself is much thicker than normal. It is believed that this is caused by a genetic mutation. Research is still being done to determine the role of high blood pressure, physical activity, and obesity.
- ♥ **Restrictive cardiomyopathy:** The heart becomes stiff and cannot fill efficiently during diastole, the period of the heartbeat when the chambers fill with blood. This condition is rare in the United States and other industrialized nations. It is the least understood of the cardiomyopathies. Fortunately, it is a rare disease, since we have few options for treatment other than transplant.

Cardiomyopathy can also be caused by drug and alcohol use, a viral infection, or hypertension; it can also be idiopathic, meaning there is no clear cause.

Alcohol use, specifically, can lead to dilated cardiomyopathy. Recent studies have shown that alcoholic women are more likely to develop cardiomyopathy than alcoholic men. Even though women in the studies consumed less than 60% of the total amount of alcohol that men did, the incidence of cardiomyopathy was equal in the two groups. This leads us to believe that the smooth muscle of a woman's heart is affected more seriously by alcohol than that of a man's heart.

What to Look For

CHF can show up in many ways. The most common symptom is fluid retention of some sort, in the limbs or the lungs. There can be swelling of the feet and legs, difficulty breathing or catching your breath, fatigue, weakness, or difficulty breathing while lying on your back. In a more advanced state, it may be necessary to sleep with several pillows or sitting up in order to breathe. If you smoke, have a history of hypertension, diabetes, or heart attack, you are at increased risk.

Testing

If you notice any of these symptoms, especially if you have the risks factors mentioned, be certain to have your physician evaluate your symptoms. The best way to treat heart failure is to prevent its occurrence by treating the underlying disease process. There are several tests available to diagnose CHF. The most common is an echocardiogram. Your doctor may also order blood tests, an exercise stress test, or other imaging tests.

Exercise echocardiography and Nuclear Imaging

Technology has made marvelous strides in the assessment and diagnosis of disease, not just of the heart but of all systems in the body. Two of the most useful and widely-used tests in cardiology are stress echocardiography and structural abnormalities.

Stress echocardiography has proven very effective in diagnosing heart disease. Where other tests seem to be most useful for men, studies show that stress echocardiography is more reliable for women than a regular electrocardiogram. It is a noninvasive and relatively simple test. It uses basically the same technology as ultrasounds do for pregnancies.

Exercise electrocardiography provides information about heart size, pumping strength, damage to the heart muscle, valve problems, blood-flow patterns, and structure abnormalities. It is particularly useful in diagnosing valve problems and is used frequently for this purpose.

You will be asked to exercise on a treadmill for a set amount of time based on age and other factors. After you have finished, you will immediately be "scanned." You will be asked to lie down (which will be a welcome break after all that exercise) and a special conductive jelly will be spread on your chest area. This jelly helps amplify the sound signals. A small wand will be waved over your chest area and a signal sent to a TV monitor. The wand sends sound waves into your chest. The sound waves bounce back when they hit the structure of the heart, and this "bounced back" wave is the image displayed on the monitor. It is painless and harmless, so much so that this test is used frequently in pregnancies, even at early gestations. You will be able to see everything the doctor sees as he is scanning your heart.

Nuclear imaging sounds scary. After all, we are conditioned to avoid radiation and realize that large doses are fatal. Merely the word "nuclear" is enough to put off just about anyone. However, though radioactive material is used in this procedure, the amount is so small that is poses less threat than a simple x-ray. The technology is so sensitive that it can read a "signal" from a miniscule amount of radioactive material.

Nuclear imaging has made great strides in giving us very accurate and specific diagnoses with respect to heart disease. It shows actual heart function and blood flow through the system. It can give information about chamber size, pumping abilities of the heart, blood flow to the heart muscle itself, and blood flow to the lungs. There are many types of tests, each with a different sensitivity and focus. The most common are MUGA scans and perfusion scans. To make things just a bit more complicated, perfusion scans come in several flavors as well: technetium or sestamibi scans and thallium scans.

A MUGA scan is used mostly to determine chamber size of the heart. This is an important indicator of the strength of your heart muscle.

Perfusion scans can identify heart defects, blood flow to the lungs, and the heart's pumping ability. They can not show a blockage directly but can show the results of a blockage. If you are suspected to have a blockage within your heart an angiography would be done to further illuminate the severity and location.

The test, again, is painless, and complications are rare. It is possible to have a reaction to the radionuclides that are injected into the bloodstream, but this is not common and there are drugs that can reverse the effects immediately. Basically, the doctor will inject a trace amount of the radioactive material, or radionuclides, into your bloodstream. As these radionuclides travel through your body a sensitive camera picks up their path, which creates a surprisingly detailed image of the functioning heart. Like the echocardiography, you will be able to view the images on a monitor. Some tests involve exercising prior to being scanned, others don't. It depends on the purpose for the exam and the specific information your doctor is seeking.

These tests can be life-saving in that they provide accurate, specific information about the function of one's heart. They are especially important for women, as some of the more "traditional" tests do not reveal heart disease in women as successfully. If your doctor has any suspicion of heart disease, and it is not revealed on an EKG, insist on further testing.

Treatment

There are many medications aimed at improving heart function when it is in failure. If you are interested in the specifics of these drugs, please see the sidebar to this section. Fortunately, these drugs are effective at slowing the progression of CHF. They will be enough treatment for the majority of women. However, for a handful of those with end-stage CHF, the only treatment option may be a heart transplant.

Sarah's Story

My eyes are heavy, and even though I want to open them, it feels like there are weights holding closedown my eyelids. I would like to move my arms, but I can't. I feel panic starting to rise in my throat. I'm not sure where I am or why I can't move. Then, I hear a soft voice telling me to relax. I am in the recovery room after surgery. My body will wake up slowly. Then I remember. A flood of relief, not only because I know where I am but because I survived the surgery. I will see my son again. I will see my family.

I'm sure I drifted in and out for a time. I have lost track of the minutes, but the nurse is here telling me that I am ready to be moved to a room in the CCU. She tells me that my husband is there and that in a few hours they will remove the tubes in my throat and turn off the respirator.

I don't feel sore like I thought I would, but I imagine that will catch up to me. I don't think they can crack your chest open and immobilize your heart without producing any ill effects. Actually, the doctor told me that the recovery time will be about six weeks, maybe a bit longer because the surgery can be more difficult for women. I'm so glad to have survived the surgery that I promise God I will do everything I can to recover quickly and to keep my life on the straight and narrow. I know the doc told me only a small percentage of surgeries have complications, but I'm still so happy to be conscious that I would promise anything to express my thanks to the angels watching over me.

The nursing assistants wheel me down the hall to my home away from home for the next week or so. My eyes still don't want to focus, but I can see the blurry image of my husband standing in the doorway. His face shows a curious mix of happiness and worry. I can't talk until they remove the tubes, but I give him my best thumbs-up. He takes my hand and kisses my forehead. He must sense my concern for Josh, because he tells me right away that Josh is with Mom and doing well. She is spoiling him with McDonald's and a new space ranger toy. I realize how perceptive yet resilient our little ones are, and I am thankful that he can be distracted from some of the scary feelings he must be having.

HEART FAILURE—SUMMARY

- ♥ Risk factors
- ♥ Congenital heart disease
- ♥ Valvular disease
- ♥ Heart muscle disease
- ♥ Coronary artery disease
- ♥ High blood pressure

Symptoms in Women
- ♥ Shortness of breath
- ♥ Fatigue with exertion
- ♥ Shortness of breath when lying down
- ♥ Swelling of the feet, legs, and/or trunk
- ♥ Palpitations
- ♥ Syncope

Testing
- ♥ Echocardiogram
- ♥ Chest x-ray
- ♥ Cardiac catheterization
- ♥ Nuclear scans of the heart
- ♥ Exercise stress test
- ♥ Electrocardiogram (EKG)

Treatment
- ♥ Positive inotropic medications.
- ♥ Vasodilators
- ♥ Diuretics
- ♥ Beta-blockers
- ♥ Anticoagulants
- ♥ Cardiotonics
- ♥ Heart transplant

Prognosis
- ♥ Varies considerably depending on severity of failure

Prevention
- ♥ Avoidance of primary heart disease

The Beating Heart

Most days we never give thought to our heart and its steady beat. If it is behaving as it should, it thumps on reliably, and we take little notice. When our beloved enters the room, we may feel it quicken or leap. If we are stimulated by a particularly exciting piece of music, we may notice its dance. For the most part, though, I liken heartbeat to how I feel about my car. As long as it starts easily and runs smoothly, I don't give a second thought to what is going on under the hood. However, when it starts to clank or clang, I begin to obsess over what might be wrong. The same holds true for our hearts. As long as they are working, we don't think about them. When they begin to protest and make their presence known, we become concerned.

The clanks and clangs of the heart can be benign, as they are in the case of some palpitations, or they can be more troublesome, as they are with arrhythmias. Let's take a look at the brains of the heart, the electrical system, which controls its fascinating beat.

The Brains: The Nodes and His-Purkinje

The tissues of your heart are actually electrified, not much different than you are when you put your finger in a light socket. Elaborately-timed electrical impulses that reverberate through the muscle create the beat of your heart.

The electrical impulse starts in the sinus node and spreads through the atria to the AV node (a group of specialized muscle fibers designed to receive and transmit electrical signals) and finally the ventricles. The sinus node can be considered the natural pacemaker, as it sets the pace for the beats. Each heartbeat is approximately one second. Unlike other muscle cells, the cardiac cells can start their own electrical impulses and contractions. In essence, the heart has its own "brain." It can continue beating for an impressive length of time even after being removed from the body.

This electrical signal must travel an exact path at a measured speed. Difficulties with this system could manifest as an exceptionally fast or slow heart rate, or arrhythmia.

Hour of Death

According to the American Heart Association, men with fatal congestive heart failure are most likely to die at either midnight or near dawn, but women are most vulnerable just near dawn. Researchers believe the reason lies in the daily biological ebb and flow of hormone levels and body processes known as circadian rhythm.

There are other interesting things to note about your heartbeat. First, it is typically faster in women than men, even at rest. As you might suspect if you watch your husband napping on the couch on a Sunday afternoon, a woman's heart takes longer to relax than a man's. This might be true emotionally, but it is physiologically true as well. The exact causes for this are not known yet. Their discovery may lead to yet another leap in the treatment of heart disease in women.

Also, the heartbeat can be indication of an illness. It can be elevated due to fever, acute illness, anxiety, or anemia. Hyperthyroidism and heart defects or disease are other possible causes for an elevated heart rate. Finally, abnormal connections between arteries and veins can also cause an in increase in heart rate.

Surprisingly, a heartbeat is not the steady, plodding pulse we typically think of. Misia Landau, in the March 8, 2002, *Focus*, tell us, "There is a startling rhythm beneath the steady pulse, more like a jazz riff than a metronome." In fact, our hearts are the healthiest when they are the "bounciest" and most resilient. She also tells us, "It is the sickest hearts that may beat in the steadiest and most predictable fashion."

Women have an innate desire for and need of the rhythm of their heart. They have used it to calm a crying baby with a lullaby or entertain a restless toddler with a simple song. You can recognize a mother of an infant by the hypnotic way she shifts her weight from foot to foot, swaying to an internal rhythm designed to soothe her baby.

When the beat of a woman's heart goes wrong, it throws off her entire center of being. As an illustration of this, women are 30% more likely than men to die of an arrhythmia. Hazrat Inayat Kahn said, "What makes us feel drawn to music is that our whole being is music; our mind and our body, the nature in which we live, the nature that has made us, all that is beneath and around us, it is all music. We are close to all this music and live and move and have our being in music." This is especially true for women and is the reason they are so vulnerable to disturbances in their heart rate. Pay attention to the beat of your heart. It is uniquely you.

Palpitations and Arrhythmias

Palpitations are common in the general population, more so in women than men. They can be caused by caffeine, fear, stress, or medication. One can have palpitations but not have any abnormality in the actual rhythm of the heart itself. These palpitations are considered harmless and typically resolve themselves quickly. If they become annoying or frequent, bring them to your doctor's attention. Otherwise, you can chalk them up to one of your body's many mysteries.

They can also be an indicator of a more serious underlying problem such as an arrhythmia. Arrhythmias can have minor impacts or major impacts, such as sudden death. If you hear of a person "dropping dead" of a heart attack, it is most likely from an arrhythmia known as ventricular tachycardia.

There are four basic types of arrhythmia: conduction-system abnormalities, slow heartbeats (bradycardia), irregular heartbeats, and fast heartbeats (tachycardia). Let's look at each one and what they mean for your heart.

Postural Orthostatic Tachycardia Syndrome (POTS)
When this syndrome was first observed, the sufferers were thought to be insane. We have come along way since that time. It is a disease primarily, though not exclusively, of females and has been observed to be passed from mother to daughter. POTS is diagnosed when a patient's heartbeat increases more than 30 beat per minute after standing up. This increase must happen within 5 minutes. When a person stands, their body automatically constricts their blood vessels. This helps to maintain one's blood pressure in spite of gravity. If this system breaks down, as it does in POTS, blood pools in places where it should be flowing rapidly. The heart then has to work many times harder than normal to get the blood moving again. Longstanding POTS can have many devastating effects such as memory impairment, poor balance, numbness, and it has been linked to chronic fatigue syndrome as well.

♥ **Conduction-system abnormality:** The heart conducts "electricity" from the upper-right chamber, through the middle of the heart, to the lower chambers through the special conducting fibers. Slowing or interruption of this conduction is called a conduction-system abnormality.

♥ **Slow heartbeat:** Any time the heart rate drops below 50 beats per minute, the rate is considered to be slow. However, the circumstances must be taken into consideration. During sleep, for example, it is not unusual for the heart rate to go as low as the 30s or 40s.

♥ **Irregular heartbeat:** This disorder can manifest in the form of extra beats (extrasystole), premature beats, or chaotic beating (atrial fibrillation). Atrial fibrillation is the most common. There are over 2 million Americans with this abnormality and 160,000 new cases occurring annually. It occurs more frequently with age.

Atrial fibrillation is prone to cause palpitations and send the heart racing to a rate of 300 or 400 beats a minute. If this rapid heartbeat continues for an extended time, it may lead to dilated cardiomyopathy. The most serious consequence is the risk of a blood clot forming in an atrium. Because vessels are not actively contracting, blood may not be propelled normally through the atria. This lack of normal propulsion motion predisposes to clotting. If a clot dislodges and travels to the brain, a stroke can occur. If it blocks an artery in some other region, the interrupted blood flow can lead to damage elsewhere.

Fast heartbeats: Tachycardia is defined as a lasting heart rate above 100 beats per minute while resting. It is a common problem for many women and can have many causes. It can also be exasperated by hormonal fluctuations, particularly premenstrually.

What to Look For

The symptoms for these arrhythmias vary widely, ranging from nausea to palpitations to sudden death. The key to diagnosing arrhythmias is to watch for changes in your heart rate or overall well-being that are out of character for you. For example, some people are extremely sensitive to their heartbeat, and they may feel every palpitation every time one happens. Because palpitations are common in all of us, this is not really a cause for concern. If you rarely feel palpitations and suddenly feel them frequently or they seem particularly fast or hard, you should bring them to the attention of your doctor.

Lightheadedness, dizziness, and passing out comprise a "constellation" of symptoms that may occur with an arrhythmia. All of them in combination would certainly indicate that there could be a problem with your heart rhythm. However, there are many reasons that any one of these could occur. Again, watch for changes in your overall health—anything alarming or constant.

A Different Kind of Rhythm

Researchers have found that the heart and liver have their own routine, their own rhythm, per se, over a 24-hour cycle. The cycles dictate metabolism, digestion, and blood pressure. (Storch 2002)

Testing

Electrocardiograms come in two flavors. One test can be performed in a doctor's office and the other portable type, often called a Holter monitor, can be done at home and work. An EKG is the most common test used to diagnose an abnormal heart rhythm. It traces the electrical rhythms of the heart and gives an excellent picture of how the conduction system is working.

Prior to an EKG, your doctor will conduct an extensive history and physical with you. He or she will ask many questions about your health history and overall current wellbeing. It is important to disclose any symptoms you think may be playing a factor as well as health habits and family history of heart disease.

Today, there is a rapidly-evolving field called electrophysiologic study, or EPS. It is similar to cardiac catheterization, except that in this case the monitors are electrical sensors that detect electrical impulses and monitor the heart rhythm at a detailed level. This test is commonly used after a person has been revived from a cardiac collapse. It can also be helpful in determining rhythm problems that are difficult to diagnose by other means.

Treatment

Again, treatments will vary with the person and the diagnosis. There are many, many medications available to treat arrhythmias. The options can be quite bewildering and the details of each are beyond the scope of this book. There are four major classes of drugs, depending on how they affect the electrical system of the heart. Your doctor will likely choose one of the drugs from these classes should he or she determine that medication is a viable route.

Cardioversion is an "electrical" therapy. In cardioversion, a patient will likely be lightly sedated. The heart is then "shocked" with an electrical impulse, which will hopefully put it back into its regular beat. Currently, portable defibrillators are being carried by medics, police officers, and even airplane staff for emergency situations. They are programmed to read the patient's heart rhythm and provide just the right amount of shock at exactly the right time to put the heart back into a "regular" rhythm.

Pacemakers are a surgical option. They are used most frequently with bradycardia. The modern pacemakers are not sensitive to microwaves and other phenomena as they were in the past, and the batteries can now last longer than ten years. The electronics are such that they only generate

Implanting a Pacemaker

Today, pacemaker implantation is a day surgery. The procedure is performed under mild sedation. The patient is not put to sleep. The surgeon will make an incision just below the collarbone about 2 inches long. Pacer wires are inserted into a vein under the collarbone and into the heart. The pacemaker itself is about 1/2 an inch deep and 11/2 inches wide. It is connected to the pacer wires and inserted into the incision and under the skin. The skin is then closed and the patient it able to leave the hospital the same day, or possibly the next. After a week, the patient may resume their prior activities without any limitations. Modern pacemakers can now be checked over the phone. They patient places a device and a magnet over the pacemaker and it transmits a signal over the phone that can be interpreted at the doctor's office.

stimulation when the heart requires it. What once was a marvel of modern medicine is now considered an almost "routine" surgery.

PALPITATIONS AND ARRHYTHMIAS—SUMMARY

Risk Factors
- ♥ Excessive caffeine or alcohol intake
- ♥ Hormonal fluctuations
- ♥ Underlying illness
- ♥ Previous heart attack
- ♥ Heart murmur

Testing
- ♥ History and physical
- ♥ Electrocardiogram
- ♥ Exercise tolerance testing
- ♥ Long-term monitoring
- ♥ Electrophysiologic studies

Treatment
- ♥ Lifestyle changes
- ♥ Treatment of underlying illness
- ♥ Medication
- ♥ Cardioversion
- ♥ Pacemaker
- ♥ Radiofrequency ablation

Prognosis
- ♥ Women tend to fare less well than men.
- ♥ Women are at higher risk for sudden cardiac death.

Prevention
- ♥ Maintain healthy weight.
- ♥ Eat healthy diet.
- ♥ Exercise regularly.
- ♥ Don't smoke.
- ♥ Reduce caffeine and alcohol intake.
- ♥ Have regular checkups.

Sarah's Story

After seven LONG days in the hospital, I was finally discharged, and I was right—the pain did catch up to me. There were times the center of my chest felt like it was going to implode, and the incision is hideous. I'm worried about never feeling comfortable with my husband seeing it or touching it. The doctor says that it will fade with time, but it is the entire length of my chest! By the time I left the hospital, the sharp pain had mostly subsided, but I tired so easily I could barely walk the length of the hall without resting. It is a frustrating feeling for a young woman used to chasing after a toddler.

The physical therapist and rehabilitation staff at the hospital were excellent. They set me up with diet plans, exercise plans, and lots of support. Three times a week I am taking a rehabilitation class at the hospital. The classes are grouped by age, so the other men and women are near my age and are able to offer a lot of support. Often after class, we head down to the cafeteria for a "healthy" snack and some time to vent. It is very helpful to be around people experiencing the same frustrations and anxieties. They are all in a similar stage of life and can understand the stresses that I am facing.

Speaking of stress, the doctor says that things will have to change in my life if I am going to make the best of this surgery. It is possible for this bypass to become blocked again. If I am to avoid that I need to keep my diet and exercise in line but also watch out for my mental and emotional health. He had me keep a diary of a few typical days in my life and it soon became clear, after writing down every activity for the day, that there was simply too much going on in my life. He didn't have to work hard to convince me that I needed to rearrange my priorities. For one, going back to my old job is out. The problem is not so much that I can't do it physically, but that I don't want to do it emotionally. When I go back to work, I want to be at a job with a company that understands family obligations. I want to do work that is fulfilling for reasons other than a paycheck. I am going to take some time to examine my goals and find work that is more in line with where I want to be in life.

Josh had some difficulty at first. He had a lot of questions about the surgery. He wanted to know if he could get a "bad heart" or if Daddy could die. We have spent some time talking about the concept of death, but most importantly, we are giving him as much reassurance as we can that my health problem is not "catchy" and that he did not cause it. I think with time and a consistent schedule, he is regaining some feeling of safety and normality.

My husband is a different story. This seems to have impacted him in ways that I can't fully understand. He is not willing to talk much about what he is experi-

encing. He seems frightened to touch me, as though I might break. He hasn't asked about sex, even though I have indicated that I feel ready. He waits on me hand and foot. He rarely goes out with his friends and spends as much time helping around the house as he can. Don't get me wrong, I am grateful for the help, but I am also worried about how he sees me now. I have always been an independent person, and I don't want him to see me as an invalid whom he has to care for.

One of the women in my rehab class thinks that I shouldn't look a gift horse in the mouth. Her husband has thrown himself headlong into work. He is working harder and longer than ever before. He hired part-time help to come to the house for cooking and cleaning. She says it feels like he is distancing himself from her in case she dies. She hates thinking that he sees her as having one foot in the grave. She made us all laugh last week with her ideas about invigorating their relationship. She has already lost weight, so now she is going to wear short skirts and dye her hair. She even joked about getting a breast augmentation. She says she'll do anything she can to get his attention and let him know that she is alive, well, and not going anywhere.

I guess in the end we are all affected, and we all react differently. My mom still believes time heals all wounds. In the case of the massive scar on my chest, that is true. I hope it is true for the emotional scars that my loved ones are struggling with as well.

Gatekeepers

As we age emotionally, we have a tendency toward one of two moods: brittleness or flaccidity. If you were to canvas a nursing home or retirement community, you would find caricatures of both styles. You may encounter the elderly widower who has a predetermined schedule and follows it religiously every day, or perhaps you would come across a frail, stooped figure that struggles to find the right words, let alone independence. This same type of aging process happens within the heart as well, particularly the valves of the heart. The two most common types of valve failure are hardening of the valve leaflets (stenosis) and weakening of the valves (regurgitaiton).

As you may remember from our earlier discussion, the heart has four chambers. These chambers are separated by four valves, the mitral, tricuspid, aortic, and pulmonary. The atria of the upper heart receive blood from the veins and the ventricles on the bottom and pump blood into the arteries. When the ventricles relax (diastole), pressure decreases, the mitral and tricuspid valves open, and blood flows from the atria to the ventricles. The aortic and pulmonary valves are closed, preventing blood from returning into the atria. When the heart contracts (systole), the pressure forces blood through the aortic and pulmonary valves into the atria. The other two valves close to prevent blood from flowing back into the ventricles.

The valves create a one-way movement of the blood and keep blood flowing under pressure in the right direction. You might think of a valve as a faucet, mechanical and rigid. However, your heart valves are actually made of "leaflets," fluid sheets of tissue. These leaflets billow and dance like bed sheets blowing on a clothesline. Their remarkable construction allows them to seal tightly when closed and open easily when pressure is applied.

Valvular Heart Disease

Finally, Some Good News!
"Long-term data from the Framingham Heart Study indicates that during the past 50 years, the incidence of heart failure has declined among women while remaining the same among men, and that survival has improved for both sexes...Although heart failure is not epidemic, it is an enormous problem," Dr. Levy says. "It is a leading cause of hospitalization and remains a lethal condition," he adds. "Indeed, these data underscore the complexity of the epidemic and our inability to understand with confidence whether—let alone why—the epidemiology of heart failure is changing." (Levy et al. 2002)

The valves can fail, either through stenosis and regurgitation or other conditions, such as mitral valve prolapse (MVP) or congenital problems. MVP in particular is of concern to women, as 6-10% of young women have this condition. It is particularly evident in thin young women. However, most cases of MVP are harmless. Only 15% of those with MVP will suffer symptoms significant enough to require evaluation and consideration of valve surgery.

When a valve ages or becomes "tight," it is said to be stenotic. The problem with this condition is that it forces the blood through a smaller opening, which causes the heart to work much harder. Symptoms for this disease will vary depending on which valve opening is affected.

Regurgitation happens when the valve leaflets do not seal properly, either because they have become stiff with age or they have become weakened. When the valves do not seal tightly, blood backs up into the chambers of the heart and, again, increases the workload and the heart functions inefficiently.

What to Look For

For some, valve problems create no symptoms at all. Many won't know they have a problem until it is caught by an alert physician during a physical examination. Others may experience shortness of breath, dizziness, lung congestion, chest pain, and/or irregular heart rhythms. The symptoms may escalate over years and years and require no treatment at all. In other cases, they may come on rapidly and escalate quickly, requiring urgent medical care.

Testing

Echocardiogram and angiography are the two tests most likely to be used after heart valve problems have been identified.

Echocardiography is basically an ultrasound of the heart. It gives a clear visual picture of blood flow in the heart and images of the actual valves themselves. It is an accurate test for diagnosing valvular problems. It is a painless test, much like receiving an ultrasound during pregnancy.

Sex and Known Heart Disease

Believe it or not, having sex may reduce the risk of heart disease. It seems that men can reduce the risk of a major heart attack or stroke by having sex three or four times a week. Whether you are happy about this news or not, what happens with sex after a heart attack? Is it safe? How soon is too soon? Is it safe at all with known heart disease?

The answers to these questions are not nearly as complicated as you might think. If you can tolerate the exertion of walking two flights of stairs briskly, you can most likely tolerate the physical stress of sex. These activities cause about the same amount of physical exertion. Of course, much depends on the actual form of your disease and your doctor's recommendations. However, even after a major heart attack, most people are able to have sex within a couple of weeks, but emotional adjustments may be a different story.

Heart disease may have already caused numerous changes in your life, and sex has a way of complicating matters. The most important thing to keep in mind is to take it slow. Don't push yourself to have sex if you don't feel ready. There are many ways to be intimate with your significant other, sex being only one of them. You may be experiencing a lot of fear and anxiety about having sex in the face of heart disease or in the aftermath of a heart attack. You may be worried that you will experience another attack or worsen your symptoms. The best thing you can do for yourself is acknowledge these emotions and fears and do your best to accept them. They will likely be with you for awhile. I liken it to learning to ride a bike. It was scary at first and hardly seemed worth the risk, but once you took the leap of faith that you can make that bike stay upright on two wheels, the rest is a piece of cake. But you couldn't do it until you were good and ready, no matter who was watching, teasing, or cajoling.

You need to maintain open communication with your partner as well. It is likely that they are experiencing a significant amount of anxiety themselves. They may feel that they don't want to do anything to exacerbate your condition. Talk with them candidly and create an open forum where the two of you can express your anxieties without judgment. This, in itself, is one of the most intimate things a couple can do.

Illness has a way of closing one set of doors but opening another. Use this opportunity to be vulnerable with your partner in ways that you haven't been in the past. Your relationship will be the richer for it and eventually sex will be the expression of the mutual trust and warmth that has developed.

Catheterization and angiography are additional options. There are several different types and techniques. Basically, dye is injected into a blood vessel through a catheter so that the circulatory system can be more clearly visualized on x-ray film. These tests provide very clear images of the heart, valves, and blood flow and are of immense value in diagnosing valve problems.

Treatment

Depending on the severity of your valvular disease, you may or may not require medication. Valve disease reduces the heart's ability to pump efficiently. This can lead to symptoms of heart failure. The good news is there are many medications that can help, including digitalis, diuretics, and vasodilators. It may also be necessary to use an anticoagulant medication to prevent blood clots from forming.

There are three basic treatments for advanced valvular disease: balloon dilatation, valve repair, and valve replacement. Balloon dilatation, or balloon valvuloplasty, is used most often to treat pulmonary or mitral stenosis. A small catheter is threaded into the heart through blood vessels. When the catheter is properly placed in the valve in question, the balloons are inflated. This enlarges the valve opening and allows more blood to flow freely through the opening.

In certain cases of valve disease, a repair will be necessary. The form and technique used will vary depending on which valve is implicated and the extent of the disease. If it is possible to repair the valve versus having a replacement, the results will likely be longer lasting and you may not require additional medications after the surgery.

In other cases, a total replacement is necessary. There are many types of prosthetic valves that can be used. Some are mechanical and constructed from metal and other synthetic materials. Some are called bioprosthesis—these valves are made from animal or human tissue. The animal tissue is usually taken from a pig's heart valve or the lining of a cow's heart. The human tissue valves are donated, and the benefit is that they do not cause rejection.

VALVULAR HEART DISEASE—SUMMARY

Risk Factors
- ♥ Coronary disease or heart attack
- ♥ Aging
- ♥ Congenital damage
- ♥ Scoliosis or other skeletal problems.

Symptoms in Women
- ♥ Shortness of breath
- ♥ Lung congestion
- ♥ Chest pain
- ♥ Irregular heart rhythms

Testing
- ♥ Physical examination
- ♥ Echocardiogram
- ♥ Angiography

Treatment
- ♥ Medications such as digitalis, diuretics, or vasodilators, as well as anti-coagulants
- ♥ Catheterization
- ♥ Surgical valve repair
- ♥ Valve replacement

Prognosis
- ♥ Women are at higher risk for mitral valve prolapse.
- ♥ Symptoms typically develop slowly over many years, sometimes as long as 20-30.

Prevention
- ♥ Avoidance of primary heart disease
- ♥ Proper diet
- ♥ Avoidance of diet drugs and extreme diets or weight loss

Sarah's Story

It has been nearly a year since the bypass surgery, and fortunately for me, I couldn't feel any better. I believe I am happier and healthier than I was before the heart attack. A few in my rehab class have not been as fortunate.

I have been determined to make the best out of a horrible situation. This type of surgery is not something I would wish on my worst enemy. I promised myself that I would do better to care for my heart and my health. I owe it to myself and to my family, especially my son.

Many things have changed within the past year. I have watched Josh gain a year. He has outgrown some of his "aggression" and is concentrating better in school. He is still feisty, but he seems to be more considerate of others, particularly his friends and other children. I would like to attribute this to the additional time I am spending with him. We've been talking more and I've been trying to model behaviors that I would like him to pick up. I couldn't put a price on the time I've had with him over the last few months.

I have not maintained an "exercise program" in any formal sense. I get my exercise around the house, in the garden, walking with Josh, playing catch. I also have taken up swimming with a Master's group in the winter and play softball in the summer. I take the stairs where I can rather than the elevator. I walk or ride my bike where I can for errands. I didn't join a gym or hire a trainer. I just try to make my life as active as possible. We have been hiking and camping and fishing, too. Whatever we can do to stay off the couch, away from the TV, and out of the house. It is even better that we can do many of these things as a family.

Diet was a real struggle for me in the beginning. I spent a lot of time agonizing over the things that I couldn't eat. After a time of torturing myself, I decided that things I could eat vastly outweighed the things I couldn't. Also, when I was able to take up more activity and do things I enjoyed, my cravings for sugars and fats declined. We have a running joke in the house about my George Foreman grill, which has become my best friend, along with my "light" versions of everything. My friends from rehab class have even started recipe swaps. My family can't tell the difference between "healthy" and not. In fact, I think they prefer the newer foods I have been preparing.

Last but not least, I have started a part-time job working for a non-profit agency that raises money for people who can't afford health insurance. Lucky for me, we had good insurance and the medical bills were manageable. There are so many that are financially devastated when an illness hits. Even worse, they are denied care that they need because they don't have insurance to pay for it. I am able to fit my hours in around Josh's schedule. Of course, I am not paid at the same level of my old position, but we have been able to cut out many expenses, such as wardrobe, travel, child care, that were a part of the old job to make up the difference. Regardless of pay, I wouldn't go back. I love knowing that the work I do makes a difference.

I guess the most important realization I made was that I DESERVE to be healthy. I deserve to eat right. My body deserves to be exercised. My mind deserves to be exercised. My heart deserves to be loved and to beat. I can't say that all of the nagging problems of life have resolved themselves—they haven't. I still pay bills and wash dishes and vacuum. I detest knowing that people are starving in the world and not knowing what the world will be like in twenty years for my son. I argue with the neighbors about their speedy driving habits in our residential street, and I am guilty of harboring many ill thoughts about people that cut me off in traffic. But at the end of the day, when I tally up the good and the bad, when I detoxify and weed out what is worth stressing over and what isn't, my balance sheet comes up in the positive. Could I have made these changes prior to the heart attack? Yes, I could have, and I wish that I had. But like my mom says, "It doesn't matter where you lead the horse or how it drinks the water, only that it drinks." Thanks, Mom.

Infectious Heart

Before we go on to talk about the last disease process, pericarditis, let's talk a bit about Sarah's story. By now, you know her struggles and strengths. How different is her life from yours? How different is her heart from yours? In the final analysis, we all have common experiences that draw us together and differences that dilute the power of our interconnections. I mention this in order to caution you against reading her story too lightly. Often, as a defense mechanism, it is our nature to create differences where there are none in order to avoid facing our own frailties. Maybe Sarah's daily life is vastly different from your own: She works in an office, you work at home. She is married, you are widowed. She has children, you have grandchildren. Whatever the differences, there will be commonalities: You are both strong, tenacious, spirited. Maybe you are both frightened and exhausted. Don't let the differences cloud the reality. All women are susceptible to heart disease, some more than others. It happened to Sarah, and it can happen to you.

Great Imitators: Non-Cardiac Chest Pain

With all of our talk about chest pain and heart disease, it can be easy to read disaster into every muscle twitch. In fact, there are many causes for chest pain that are not related to heart disease. Unfortunately, they can be difficult to diagnose and they can cause a great deal of pain.

Chest pain can be mild or severe. It can occur intermittently or constantly. It may radiate from the center of the chest or be felt in the shoulder or neck. Cardiac chest pain can be elusive, but the diagnosis is complicated when we consider non-cardiac causes as well. Women of any age can have chest pain, whether it is cardiac or non-cardiac.

If you have complaints of chest pain, your doctor will rule out cardiac causes but look for non-cardiac causes as well. The esophagus lies close to the heart and therefore can be a common source of chest pain that is confused with cardiac problems. Gastroesophageal reflux disease (GERD), esophageal spasm, and muscle inflammation are some possibilities. Anxiety and panic attacks are other common causes.

Non-cardiac chest pain typically starts in the middle of the chest and is felt as a dull, burning, or pressure sensation. It does not usually radiate to the neck, arms, or shoulders. If the chest pain is linked to musculoskeletal concerns, it could be located anywhere on the chest wall. You may also have muscle and joint pains, fatigue, and trouble with sleeping.

Anxiety and panic attacks are a phenomenon of their own and deserve special mention. Typically, this type of pain will be felt as a sharp twinge and will be accompanied by a feeling of impending doom. It will be difficult to catch your breath and you may sweat profusely or have difficulty sleeping. Panic attacks are relatively common disorders and, in the worst cases, can be readily treated with antidepressants. A word of caution here, however. Do NOT let your doctor simply "brush off" chest pain as anxiety until other potential cardiac causes have been ruled out.

If it turns out that your chest pain is non-cardiac in nature, the treatment will vary with the diagnosis. GERD is commonly treated with antacids and other medications. There are some exceptionally strong, sophisticated drugs available for the most resistant cases. It is important to treat GERD, as it can also be a precursor to esophageal cancer. Musculoskeletal pains are easily treated with appropriate exercise and anti-inflammatory drugs. Anxiety and panic attacks can be treated with drugs, but counseling may be a good option to ferret out the psychological causes.

Whatever the cause for your chest pain, do not ignore the signs and symptoms. Chest pain should be taken seriously and thoroughly investigated before any diagnosis is made.

This statement is not intended to frighten you. I simply want to be certain that you take the right steps toward a healthy heart. Heart disease, for the most part, is preventable. There are many things we can do (or not do) that will lessen the chances of encountering trouble in the future. As you learned from Sarah's story, hope is a powerful force, and best of all, it is infectious. With that, let's talk a bit about pericarditis, infection of the lining of the heart.

The heart has three layers, the endocardium, myocardium, and epicardium. The myocardium is the center layer and provides the bulk of the muscle. The endocardium and epicardium are thinner protective layers. You can think of them as a sort of lubricant that keeps the heart from being damaged by constant friction and rubbing. The heart tissue and the blood vessels emerging from it are contained by a sac called the pericardium.

Under certain conditions, this sac becomes irritated, which causes inflammation. Fluid builds up between the outer and inner layers and compresses the heart, which restricts its pumping action. Constrictive pericarditis results from a thickening of the pericardium that leads to restricted movement of the heart. Cardiac Tamponade occurs when blood or fluid collects in the pericardium and causes difficulty.

What to Look For

A common symptom is sharp chest pain that is reduced by sitting up or leaning forward. This pain may radiate to the neck or back. It is different from angina because it is a stabbing pain centered directly over the heart. It is also common to have difficulty breathing, especially when lying down. Other symptoms are consistent with an infection that may happen regardless of its location in the body: Fever, sweating, dizziness, fatigue, and loss of appetite.

In most cases, the cause of the infection is never found. Fortunately, in these cases, the infection almost always clears within six weeks. There may be a connection with a viral or bacterial infection. Also, some diseases and cancers can cause conditions in the body that lead to pericarditis.

Testing

Your doctor will do a thorough examination. He or she will determine your level of pain and anxiety. They may hear a friction rub when they listen to your heart. This is the result of the two layers of the pericardium rubbing against each other.

Blood tests may reveal an increase in white blood cells due to the infection. An EKG will uncover a characteristic pattern particular to pericarditis. Echocardiograph and catheterization may also be used.

Treatment

With mild cases, rest is the best option. Your doctor may also prescribe aspirin or another nonsteroidal anti-inflammatory drug for a couple of weeks. Prednisone may occasionally be used, but it typically has side effects.

In a more severe case, demonstrating heart problems, you may be hospitalized and monitored with EKGs. It may be necessary to drain fluids from around the heart as soon as possible. If all of these remedies fail, surgery to remove the pericardium may be required. Fortunately, it is not likely one would notice any significant differences once having this lining removed.

PERICARDITIS—SUMMARY

Risk Factors
- ♥ Viruses such as coxsackie B, adenovirus, mumps, and Epstein-Barr
- ♥ Bacterial infection such as staphylococcus, haemophilus, pneumococcus, and salmonella
- ♥ Acute rheumatic fever
- ♥ Tuberculosis
- ♥ Certain drugs, such as phenytoin, procainamide, hydralazine, and minoxidil
- ♥ Diseases, such as cancer, lupus, rheumatoid arthritis, and pancreatitis
- ♥ Radiation therapy

Symptoms in Women
- ♥ Sharp or stabbing chest pain
- ♥ Difficulty breathing, particularly when lying down
- ♥ Fever
- ♥ Cough
- ♥ Sweating
- ♥ Dizziness
- ♥ Fatigue
- ♥ Loss of appetite

Testing
- ♥ Thorough physical examination
- ♥ Blood tests
- ♥ EKG
- ♥ Echocardiogram
- ♥ Cardiac catheterization

Treatment
- ♥ Rest
- ♥ Aspirin or other NSAID
- ♥ Draining of fluid accumulation around the heart
- ♥ Removal of the pericardial lining

Prognosis
- ♥ It is rarely a life-threatening condition.
- ♥ Women are more predisposed to Cardiac Tamponade than are men.

Prevention
- ♥ Avoidance of viral and bacterial infections

CHAPTER 5

Hormone-Replacement Therapy

Estrogen: The Female Advantage

The other night, my wife and I were discussing exactly how to split the household duties. We both work professional jobs that entail long hours and lots of stress. She is pregnant and feeling overwhelmed by the sheer coordination of it all. There is the baby's room to prepare, a house to clean, provisions to be made, and the list goes on. I, in my typically male obtuseness, did not clue in to the amount of pressure she was feeling. Then the famous words escaped her lips: "I just do and do and do around here, and you do NOTHING!" This wasn't a particular revelation, because we both knew that she shoulders the majority of the burden for the housekeeping and management. What got my attention was the tone and the specific words. She could have been my mother arguing with my father. My mother, a particularly hard-working woman, would occasionally engage in arguments with my father over the very same topic, and she would air the very same frustrations. It took a two-by-four over the head, but it was then that I understood that my wife's frustrations were common to women everywhere.

Over the next few weeks, I informally polled my female patients. I asked them about the pressures they feel on a daily basis. I talked with them about the division of work in their households, and I started to develop a sense of how much women really do concern themselves with the "small" details of life. By small, I do not mean unimportant. I am talking about the everyday, mundane concerns that make the world tick.

For years, researchers have looked at stress from the "fight-or-flight" angle. We discuss this same perspective throughout the book. Interestingly enough, women seem to have an innate hormonal advantage when it comes to dealing with chronic stress. It is the same hormonal advantage that protects against cardiovascular disease, the wonderful hormone known as estrogen.

Perimenopause

Technically, menopause is defined as the cessation of menstruation. Perimenopause, in that case, is the time before and after menopause. What are some of the signs of perimenopause?

1. Irregular menstrual periods
2. Hot flashes
3. Night sweats
4. Vaginal dryness
5. Difficulty sleeping
6. Mood swings

It seems that the negative effects of stress are best combated by a hormone known as oxytocin. It is not certain that women have more oxytocin than men, but they do have more estrogen, which enhances the beneficial effects of oxytocin. This hormone has come to be known as the "cuddling" or social-attachment hormone, because it is produced in prodigious amounts during childbirth and lactation and during orgasm. Its production is also stimulated by other types of pleasant touch. Researchers have linked it to bonding in animals, as well.

The powerful combination of oxytocin and estrogen supports the idea that flight or fight is not the only way to cope with stress; women also cope by "tending and befriending." Turning to relationships for moral support and nurturing the young act as stress relievers for women. This seems to refute the fight-or-flight paradigm.

Therefore, as usual, things are not as clear-cut as they might seem. The standard position that women are merely "small men" just doesn't hold, and estrogen is a key component in proving that.

For example, estrogen provides over 300 functions in a woman's body and comes in three basic forms: estradiol, estrone, and estriol. Estradiol is the main estrogen made by a woman's ovaries before menopause. Estrone is a weaker estrogen produced in the ovaries and also in fat tissue from other hormones, mainly after menopause. Estriol is the weakest of the three forms and is made from other estrogens. The amount of these estrogens in a woman's body varies greatly over the course of her menstrual cycle, as well as her lifetime.

No wonder women feel pulled in 300 different directions. All kidding aside, we know about some of the effects of estrogen, but most research has centered on the effects of lower estrogen levels. The primary effect is the cessation of one's menstrual period. When estrogen drops precipitously, the uterus is not stimulated to produce an endometrial lining, and therefore, has nothing to shed by way of a cycle. Low estrogen levels have also been blamed for—

♥ Hot flashes, night sweats, and disturbed sleep

♥ Osteoporosis

♥ Skin changes

♥ Breast changes

♥ Changes in mood or depression

♥ Loss of sexual desire

♥ Vaginal dryness and lessening elasticity of the vaginal tissue
♥ Increase in cholesterol levels

All of the effects lead to the wonderful stage of life known as menopause. I don't say "wonderful" here facetiously. For many years, science has looked at menopause as an illness to be treated. Menopause is not an illness; it is a natural cycle of life. Menopause serves an important function for women, as do the stages of puberty and the reproductive years. It is no less important, just different.

In our era of convenience and comfort, menopause is seen as a discomfort, something to be suffered through. I believe this attitude is much of what is at the root of the issues surrounding the "difficulties" of middle life. The medical field also has a tendency to view menopause as a "cause" of heart disease. Being male has never been a risk factor for heart disease, and neither is being female. Women are simply "protected" by estrogen for a period of time. Once their system stops manufacturing estrogen, that protection fades, and they become equal to men in the incidence of heart disease.

Because researchers are always quick to look for ways to "relieve suffering," many treatments have tried to mitigate the problems associated with menopause, not the least of these being hormone-replacement therapy.

Studies, Studies, Studies

Throughout the course of this book we have referenced many, many studies. Here is an overview of some of the largest.

- WISE: Women's Ischemia Syndrome Evaluation.
- Nurse's Health Study.
- WHI: Women's Health Initiative.
- HERS: Heart and Estrogen/Progestin Replacement Study.
- Framingham Heart Study.

What is HRT, Exactly?

Hormone-replacement therapy, HRT for short, is the process of introducing additional hormones, either synthetic or natural, into the body. The hormone introduced may be estrogen alone or estrogen in combination with progestin. These hormones can be taken as a pill, patch, shot, or under the tongue.

The most commonly-prescribed from of HRT is a mixture of estrogens extracted from the urine of pregnant mares. (Premarin and Prempro are the most recognizable names.) Prempro is a combination of estrogen and progestin and is the most widely-known combination therapy.

One of the primary uses for HRT has been to help reduce cholesterol. Because of the known cardioprotective effect of estrogen, doctors prescribed it in the hope of reducing the risk of heart disease. After a time, estrogen was being prescribed not only for "quality-of-life" improvements but also for physical gains, such as prevention of heart disease, osteoporosis, and Alzheimer's.

HRT and Weight Gain

There is a longstanding belief that HRT increases weight gain. However, a study published in May 2003 contradicts this position. Researchers found that women NOT taking HRT experienced more weight gain over five years than the women using hormone treatment.

If the loss of estrogen could produce all of the "negative" effects we discussed in the previous section, then surely introducing estrogen could reverse these effects. In some cases, it was as simple as that. However, unknown factors were also at play, and some of the detrimental effects of HRT are now coming to light.

Current Research

In July 2002, the Women's Health Initiative study published a portion of its results in the *Journal of the American Medical Association*. This article set the medical community on edge and sent women into their physicians' offices for advice. (WHI 2002)

This study was following 16,608 postmenopausal women that were in the 50-79 age bracket. Half were given an estrogen-plus-progestin combination pill and half were given a placebo. WHI requested that all women in the study stop taking their combination hormone replacement at approximately the five-year mark, because they had found an increased risk for breast cancer, heart attack, stroke, and blood clots. WHI felt that the known risks outweighed the known benefits (fewer fractures and colorectal cancers).

In fact, the study came to even more surprising conclusions. After one year of the treatments, there was no appreciable difference between the HRT and the placebo with respect to "quality of life," meaning that there was no statistical difference in how the two groups of women assessed general health, physical functioning, bodily pain, energy, social functioning, mental health, depression, sleep disturbances, sexual satisfaction, or symptoms associated with menopause.

Heart Attack Risk Higher on Low-Estrogen Days

A small study published in the journal *Heart* indicated that young women with heart disease are more likely to suffer a heart attack the week during or after their menstrual periods.

On one hand, this is almost intuitive, in the sense that estrogen offers a protective effect on the cardiovascular system and estrogen is at its lowest during this time period.

The study suggests that women take into consideration the menstrual cycles when scheduling heart studies. Heart disease may be missed if tested when estrogen levels are at their peak. (Lloyd et al. 2000)

Finally, in an article published in *JAMA* in May 2003, WHI researchers reported that women on combination HRT have double the risk of developing dementia (Shumaker et al. 2003). However, they were quick to caution that the results might not be applicable to younger women.

So, not only was HRT proven to be detrimental to heart health, it was shown to create little improvement in menopause symptoms. At about the same time these results were released, another large study of a similar nature released their results as well. The HERS ("Heart and Estrogen/Progestin Replacement Study") came to similar conclusions. After four years, there was no reduction in heart attacks or deaths from coronary heart disease, in spite of an average 11% decline in LDL cholesterol levels and a 10% increase in HDL levels. (Grady et al. 2002)

One more piece of bad news for the women taking HRT: a study published in April 2003 found that estrogen taken orally "caused a robust increase in CRP," while estrogen taken in the form of a patch, at nearly twice the strength of the oral doses, had no effect on CRP levels (Vongpatanasin et al. 2003). You may remember CRP from our discussion on risk factors. This is a chemical in the blood found to be responsible for inflammation that may be an indicator of heart disease.

If you add all of these risk factors together, along with the known risks for increased breast cancer, ovarian cancer, and osteoarthritis, you may wonder why HRT is still available at all. There are many, many reasons. Let's look at a few.

Pros and Cons: Weighing the Odds

There are many reasons HRT is still available, prescribed, and used. First of all, the two major studies, WHI and HERS, though eye-opening, are still studies. The results are based on population samples and statistics. There will always be discrepancies and uncertainties when reporting numbers of this type. For example, both studies were designed around an older age bracket. This has a definite impact on many factors, including prevalence of existing heart disease, activity levels, general health, etc.

The WHI study results were for estrogen/progestin combination drugs only. The results for the estrogen arm of the study are still not out. Therefore, their findings to date are only for combination HRT. There are also many different combinations, dosages, and forms. There are studies that show differences between oral versus patch forms.

Finally, individuals are just that—individual. All women have slightly different biochemical makeups that will determine their reaction to, benefit from, and risks involved with undergoing hormone-replacement therapy. There are still many reasons to use hormone replacement. This is not an issue that can be answered in a black-and-white manner.

Potential Benefits

What are some of the potential benefits? A major study done by researchers at Wake Forest University Baptist Medical Center and Tufts-New England Medical Center (Karas and Clarkson 2003) reported that the timing of hormone-replacement therapy may be a key factor in whether or not it can slow heart vessel disease. The press release from this study states: "Mounting evidence points to the conclusion that HRT can help prevent heart vessel disease—if the therapy begins around the time that the body stops making its own estrogen." Thomas B. Clarkson, D.V.M., of Wake Forest, continues, "The question may not be if estrogen helps, but

Breast Cancer and HRT
The WHI study found a statistically significant increase in breast cancer incidence, nearly 26%, in women on combination HRT.

when is the optimum time to begin therapy…The literature demonstrates that HRT has beneficial effects in inhibiting the early stages of heart vessel disease, but can have deleterious effects if initiated at older ages, when some women have already developed disease."

These researchers believe that the WHI study and the earlier observational studies came to opposing conclusions based on the age of the women being studied. They said the data they reviewed supports the theory that HRT may be helpful in younger women that do not have atherosclerosis, but that older women with advanced disease may be harmed.

Aside from the role HRT plays in heart health, there are other considerations. Research has shown that HRT does lower LDL cholesterol levels as well as the glycemic profile. This means that women would be at lower risk for diabetes, the top risk factor for heart disease. Contrary to a popular myth, HRT does not cause weight gain, either.

Finally, there are many, many studies being done to link HRT to other benefits, such as prevention of cataracts, Alzheimer-related dementia, and colon cancer. Research shows diminished numbers in women who have taken or are taking HRT.

The biggest benefit of all is the prevention of bone loss. Osteoporosis is a serious concern for all women after menopause, and HRT is known to prevent osteoporosis to a large extent.

And what about the pesky symptoms of menopause? The WHI study concluded that HRT does not have an impact on quality of life issues in general. I take a dual stance on this topic. First of all, I agree with the basic findings of the WHI study. HRT is only one factor in quality of life. Activity, basic emotional state, stress levels, and diet all impact quality of life and feelings of well-being. There are many things we talk about through the course of this book that impact heart and general health. HRT is just one. It should be looked at from a holistic perspective. Also, we know that estrogen serves innumerable functions in the female body, and many more will likely be discovered. These complex interactions simply cannot be dealt with summarily.

The other side of this coin is, again, the population sample used for the study. The WHI study provided women with HRT regardless of whether or not they actually had troublesome menopause symptoms, such as hot flashes and sleep disturbances. Therefore, a portion of the statistics regarding quality of life is based on the responses of women who had few issues to begin with.

I do not think it is possible or advisable to ignore the observational and anecdotal evidence that HRT relieves certain side effects of menopause, such as hot flashes, sleep disturbances, energy levels, etc. I have certainly seen, throughout the course of my practice, many women helped by HRT.

Evaluating Options

Menopause is not a big, bad monster hiding in the back of your closet. It is a time of freedom, independence, and maturity. Just because the potential for heart disease or osteoporosis exists does not mean that you will end up with either. None of these disease processes are inevitable, and HRT is not the only way to avoid them. There are other possible paths to take.

Let's break down a few of the issues in a clear format in order to help you make the best decision possible.

Table 5.1
Pros and Cons of Hormone-Replacement Therapy

Pro	Con	Alternative
Lowers LDL cholesterol	Increases triglycerides	Diet, statin drugs, exercise
Decreases blood-sugar levels	Increases CRP	Diet, exercise
Prevents osteoporosis	Increases risk for heart disease	Calcium supplementation, exercise, osteoporosis drugs
Decreases risk of colon cancer	Increases risk of breast cancer	
Relieves menopause symptoms		Antidepressants, herbal remedies

Hormone-replacement therapy is not the only option for relief of menopause symptoms, nor is it the only avenue to achieving the other known benefits of HRT. What are some of the other possible courses?

- ♥ **Cholesterol Levels:** We have talked throughout this book about cholesterol and its impact on your cardiovascular health. Diet is the first and most important step in balancing the cholesterol equation. Statins are a class of drugs used with great success in lowering LDL cholesterol and increasing HDL. Finally, appropriate exercise is an ever-present helpful factor.
- ♥ **Blood-Sugar Levels:** Again, we have talked extensively about insulin resistance and diabetes. Blood-sugar levels are best controlled through moderate exercise and a healthy diet.
- ♥ **Osteoporosis:** This disease is a major concern for all menopausal women. Fortunately, it is largely preventable and treatable if found early enough. Selective estrogen receptor modulators, also known as SERMS, are a class of drugs used to build bone density for women who have osteoporosis. Fosamax is not a SERM, but it is another popular and effective drug. In the line of prevention, calcium supplementation is a viable option for women

> **Soy Nuts Lower Blood Pressure**
> Postmenopausal women who ate a 2-ounce bag of soy nuts every day had a significant reduction in their blood pressure. One explanation is that the phytoestrogen in soy nuts raise the production of nitric oxide which in turn relaxes blood vessels and lowers blood pressure.
> Internal Medicine News. March 13, 2003 by Mitchel Zoler.

who have yet to develop osteoporosis. Be sure to talk to your doctor about appropriate dosages for your age and body weight. Calcium can also come in the form of dairy products and other dietary options.

Weight-bearing exercise has also proven helpful in preventing osteo-porosis.

♥ **Menopause Symptoms:** This is the trickiest area of all, because it is individual from woman to woman and diagnosis is based on one's subjective history. The effectiveness of the treatment will also be a sub-jective issue. However, there are some avenues to consider. Antidepressants have proven effective in correcting sleep disturbances and lessening hot flashes. They are also helpful in evening out emo-tional levels. There are many natural products on the market; but again, I urge you to speak with your doctor before using any of them. To date, their effects have not been proven scientifically, and the mere fact they are natural does not mean they are safe.

Making a Decision

In the end, a decision needs to be made. The question once was, "Why aren't you on hormone-replacement therapy?" Now, the question is, "Why ARE you on hormone-replacement therapy?" Physicians no longer assume HRT will be helpful or necessary. Increasingly, women are opting for other methods of relieving their symptoms and gaining the benefits traditionally attributed to HRT.

Also, the risks of HRT are not completely proven. Many, many women take hormone-replacement therapy and never develop breast cancer. Again, the risk evaluations are based on statistics, and only you and your physician can work through the risks versus benefits for your specific issues.

Questions to Consider

Aside from considering all of the alternatives to HRT, it would help to develop a risk matrix with your physician. Some questions to consider:

- ♥ Do you have a genetic predisposition to breast or ovarian cancer? Have you had a recent mammogram? A history of breast cancer or strong familial link would be a strike against HRT. You should definitely have a mammogram prior to beginning HRT.
- ♥ Do you have a strong family history of heart disease or have you been diagnosed with it? If so, HRT would not be recommended.
- ♥ Are you at high risk for osteoporosis? HRT might be a strong consideration in this case, but evaluate all of your options.
- ♥ Are menopausal symptoms interfering with the quality of your life? Have you tried other alternatives to relieving them?

In light of the recent research, my personal bias is that HRT should be taken as a last resort. If you have tried diet and lifestyle modifications and other classes of drugs, all to no avail, then it would be time to look at HRT. I no longer think it is the first resort. There are simply too many other options available.

In the end, only your doctor can help you make a medical decision that is best for you, and only you can make the final decision about what is working and what is not. Your doctor should be available to answer questions, provide laboratory tests, and assist with interpretation of their results, but you will be the only one to decide, subjectively, whether or not you are being helped by the preventions and therapies you are undertaking.

The decision about whether or not to undergo hormone-replacement therapy has always been difficult and complicated, but it is now even more so. Use the information in this chapter as a starting point in establishing a dialogue with your physician. Together, the two of you will be able to sort through the issues, risks, and benefits. Most importantly, remember that menopause is not an ending; it is a doorway into a new phase of life. Hormone-replacement therapy does not stop the aging process, nor should you try to do so. Embrace your maturity and use it to your advantage. Menopause brings unique challenges and unique gifts. Explore them and rejoice in them.

CHAPTER 6

I Am Forty. So What Do I Do Now?

The Big Picture

As we learned in the last chapter on hormone-replacement therapy, menopause brings with it many physical changes. So far, we have focused on the cardiovascular system, but our body systems work in concert. I would like to take just a few pages to discuss health issues in general.

Middle age is not an easy time for women. They are dealing with menopause and the entire host of changes it brings. Figure in the mental and emotional challenges, and women may feel they are facing an uphill battle. Many feel alone. Some treat their experiences as a very private matter. Not having experienced menopause myself, I am not in a position to evaluate or judge what the experience is like for women, but I can share information and insight that I have gained through the years of working with and advising women during this time. It is important for us to discuss some of the general health challenges that arise in middle age, as well as some of the specifics of medical care and advocating for yourself.

The medical profession is in dire trouble. Insurance companies and HMOs, though offering a vital service, have changed the face of the field. Many fine doctors are finding it impossible to maintain a private practice because they can't afford the malpractice insurance. An article in the *Las Vegas Review* talked about a nurse practitioner potentially leaving her practice due to malpractice costs. Her insurance was set to increase from $7500 a year to $50,000. A neurosurgeon on Long Island will pay about $180,000 a year in insurance premiums. Medical schools are having difficulty attracting top students because so many are choosing other fields.

In the end, the medical field will transform itself. In the meantime, all of these factors will have an effect on the type and quality of care available to consumers. It will be mostly up to you or your support system to advocate for your own care. You need to be informed, not only medically but financially as well.

Weight, Worry, and Wallet

A patient of mine told me a funny joke the other day. It went something like this: There is more money being spent on breast implants and Viagra than on Alzheimer's research. By 2020, there should be a large elderly population with perky breasts, never-ending erections and no recollection of what to do with either of them.

The story might be humorous, but it illustrates much of where we place our priorities today. It seems that we opt for the tangible benefits in the here and now while forgoing intangible future benefits. I think this also depicts the three major concerns of middle age: weight, worry, and wallet.

A study done by Sandra Pope in 2001 found that obese middle-age women have life-impacting physical limitations twice as often as women with an average weight. That may not come as a surprise, but given the increasing population of obese individuals, it is becoming a national health crisis.

This study surveyed 16,000 women between the ages of 40 and 55. The women who reported high levels of stress, certain medical problem, or inability to pay for basic necessities also reported a reduction in their capability for performing daily activities such as bathing, carrying groceries, or climbing stairs. As we know, a reduction in overall activity will be very detrimental to heart health, as well as general health. Staying active and keeping moving is one of the best things we can do to maintain our general well-being.

Women Heart Patients Unhappy with Care

A study published in *Women's Health Issues* in 2003 relayed that 57% of the women surveyed felt they had suffered a mental illness as a result of their heart disease, with 38% reporting clinical depression. These women reported feeling isolated because their family and friends could not understand the seriousness of their illness. Many felt they could not completely fulfill their pre-heart-disease roles, and their families became resentful.

Of the women who were dissatisfied with their medical care, nearly 60% said that their physicians' attitudes played a big part. They relayed that their doctors were often insensitive, rude, abrupt, and ignorant about heart disease in women. (Maruccio et al. 2003)

What's a Woman to Do?

We will discuss diet and movement in the chapter on finding balance. These are the two most important factors in maintaining your health into your "Golden Years." However, there is a host of other considerations. Let's take a look at them.

Dental Health

Like everything else, dental health is easy to take for granted until you no longer have it. A dentist will tell you that the condition of your teeth can be an indicator of your overall health. Be sure to maintain regular dental visits, floss daily, and use fluoride toothpaste. If you have teeth that need repair, be sure to get them taken care of as soon as possible. If an infection sets in, it will be painful and can be dangerous. Bacterial endocarditis, an infection in the valves of the heart, can be caused by certain dental procedures or a raging dental infection. Certain dental procedures can also trigger this infection, because a large number of bacteria enter the bloodstream, land inside the heart, and initiate an infection.

If you already have a heart condition, you will be at increased risk. It is possible to take an antibiotic prophylactically. Be sure to discuss this with your doctor and your dentist before undergoing major dental work. Also, if you have any fever after a dental procedure, contact your doctor right away.

Another thing to consider is bone loss. As your natural estrogen levels decline, you will be at risk for loss of bone density, including jawbone density. This can lead to tooth loss.

Hormonal changes can also cause your gums to become inflamed and bleed easily. You may also find that your teeth are more cavity-prone. If you notice a burning sensation or dryness in your mouth or a change in the taste of foods, let your dentist know. He will check for bone loss and/or gum disease. Catching these symptoms early can help with dental care before the problem becomes exaggerated past the point of prevention.

You should discuss calcium and vitamin-D supplements with your doctor. As usual, pay attention to your nutritional needs. Be certain to eat a wide variety of fruits and vegetables. Look at a preventive trip to the dentist as a means of taking care of yourself rather than a torture to be endured.

Injury Prevention

All of the health in the world won't help you if you engage in risk-taking behaviors. Some things to consider:
- ♥ Always use a seatbelt.
- ♥ Be a cautious, intelligent driver. NEVER, EVER drink and drive.
- ♥ Use helmets while riding a bicycle or motorcycle.
- ♥ Check your home for risks, such as loose rugs, slippery floors, and wobbly banisters.
- ♥ Check smoke detectors once a year.
- ♥ Take a CPR training course.

Medication/Substance Use

Medications should always be taken as prescribed. Even then, review your medication list with your doctor any time there are changes. Your physician and/or pharmacist should check for interactions and other side effects. We have already talked extensively about the dangers of smoking, as well as alcohol and drug abuse. Please, never mix alcohol and prescription medications. The combination can be deadly.

Sexual Behavior

No matter what your age or marital status, safe sex is an important issue. If you have multiple partners or sex with known drug users, you are greatly increasing your chances of acquiring a sexually-transmitted disease. Always use condoms with a new partner. If you have any suspicion that you might have contracted an STD, please see your physician right away. Typically, the tests are noninvasive and painless. It is better to know as soon as possible so that treatment can begin immediately. Your doctor will walk you through other precautions that may be required, such as abstaining from sex or informing your sexual partners so that they can be treated as well.

Immunizations

There are several immunizations that adults can and should take. They are cheap insurance against common and complicated illnesses.

- ♥ **Pneumococcus:** Every patient over the age of sixty-five should have a pneumococcal vaccination. Also, if you are in a high-risk group you should be vaccinated. The high-risk group includes any person with a chronic cardiac or pulmonary disease, renal, sickle cell, or Hodgkin's disease; nephrotic syndrome; complicated diabetes; multiple myeloma; lymphoma; asplenia; alcoholism; HIV; or other immune disease.
- ♥ **Influenza:** Have this shot annually after the age of sixty-five.
- ♥ **Tetanus-Diphtheria:** A booster is required every ten years.

Breast-Cancer Detection

Though we now know that coronary disease is more likely to affect you than breast cancer, we cannot ignore the dangers this cancer presents to women. Medical research has made great strides in its treatment, and early detection can mean the difference between life and death. Here are the minimum recommendations:

- **Mammography:** A mammogram is recommended at least once a year after the age of forty.
- **Breast self-exam (BSE):** BSEs are the single best way to detect breast cancer. Every woman should do a BSE at least once a month and have an annual examination performed by a physician.

Colorectal Cancer

Breast cancer is the most predominant in females. However, there are other cancers that should be routinely screened for. These guidelines are all derived from the American Cancer Society's recommendations. Beginning at age fifty, you should follow one of these five testing schedules.

- Fecal occult blood test, yearly
- Flexible sigmoidoscopy, every five years
- Fecal occult blood test, yearly, plus flexible sigmoidoscopy, every five years
- Double-contrast barium enema, every five years
- Colonoscopy, every five years

If you have any of the following risk factors for colorectal cancer, you should have more frequent examinations:

- Personal history of colorectal cancer or adenomatous polyps
- A strong family history of colorectal cancer or polyps
- A personal history of chronic inflammatory bowel disease
- A family history of hereditary colorectal cancer syndromes

Cervical Cancer

All women should begin cervical-cancer screening about three years after they begin having vaginal intercourse, but no later then the age of twenty-one. You should have a Pap smear every year.

After the age of thirty, if you have had three normal Pap tests, you can reduce the testing schedule to less every two or three years.

After the age of seventy, if you have had three normal Pap tests in a row and no history of abnormal results in ten years, you may choose to stop having cervical-cancer screening.

If you have had a total hysterectomy you do not need Pap tests unless the removal was to treat a cancer.

Endometrial Cancer

There are currently no screening recommendations for endometrial cancer other than to be aware of the symptoms, such as abnormal bleeding or spotting. If you have or are at a high risk for hereditary nonpolyposis colon cancer, you should have an annual screening with an endometrial biopsy beginning at the age of thirty-five.

Skin Cancer

You should have a complete skin check by a physician or dermatologist every three years until the age of forty. After forty, it is important to have a check every year. Check your own skin monthly for any of the following symptoms:
- A lump that may be small, smooth, pale, waxy, or red, which may be bleeding or crusted over
- A flat patch on the skin that might be red, rough, dry, or scaly
- A lump or patch that grows or changes color or shape
- A sore that does not heal
- An itchy lump or patch

Osteoporosis

If you are postmenopausal and have sustained a fracture, you should have a bone-mineral-density scan to determine the severity of osteoporosis.

If you are younger than sixty-five AND if you have one or more risk factors, you should have a baseline screening test done. If no new symptoms or risk factors develop, a screening should be performed every two to three years. The risk factors are a personal history of fractures as an adult, Caucasian ethnicity, impaired eyesight despite adequate correction, and a history of alcoholism.

Finding Quality Care

One of the most important decisions you will make is selecting a primary-care physician. These family doctors will be the front line in your healthcare. The best-case scenario is to choose a family physician whom you have a good rapport with and who is well-qualified, then stay with that doctor as long as possible. They will then be familiar with you, your personality, and your medical history. You may see other doctors or specialists.

Choosing a doctor is one of the most important decisions anyone can make. The best time to make that decision is while you are still healthy and have time to really think about all your choices. If you have no doctor or are thinking of changing doctors, the following ideas may help you find a doctor who is right for you.

Make a List

It is obvious that you want a well-trained, competent, friendly doctor. You will be establishing, hopefully, a life-long relationship. If you doctor knows you well, he or she will be able to help you prevent health problems and manage anything that comes up. There are some key things to look for, but you may not find everything you want in one doctor. Make a list of the characteristics that are most important to you and rank your list of doctors accordingly. Don't forget your gut instinct. Often the most important factor is that you feel comfortable with your chosen physicians.

- ♥ **Board certification:** These doctors have extra training after medical school to become specialists in their chosen field of medicine. Your best choice would be a certified family-practice physician.
- ♥ **Rapport:** Choose a doctor that listens to you carefully and answers all of your questions.
- ♥ **Financial considerations:** Check office policies on financial arrangements. Is payment required upfront? What insurance does the office accept? Do they accept Medicare?
- ♥ **Location:** Is the office in a convenient location?
- ♥ **Lab Work:** How does the office handle lab work? If it is handled in a separate lab, where is that lab located?
- ♥ **Hospital affiliation:** If you have a preference, choose a doctor that works with the hospital of your choice.
- ♥ **Call group:** Does the doctor work with a group of other doctors? If so, do they have equally strong reputations? You may be asked to see one of these doctors if your primary doctor is away for any reason.

Make a Selection

Once you have ranked the issues that are most important to you, ask for referrals. Check with your family, friends, coworkers, and other health professionals. Set a goal to create a list of at least three doctors from which to choose. You will want to interview each one and see where each fits into your rankings. If you have a managed care plan, you may be limited to doctors on the insurance company's list. Many communities and hospitals also have doctor-referral lines, as do the local chapters of the American Medical Association. Once you have narrowed down your list, set up appointments to interview each doctor.

As we all know, a doctor's time is in high demand. It is rare that we are able to sit and chat without inconveniencing all of the patients that will follow later in the day. Typically, our schedules are packed from early morning to early evening. When you set up your interview appointment, be clear with the scheduler what you are hoping to accomplish so they can allow enough time for the appointment.

Before you go, make a list of questions for each physician. This will save time and help you better organize your search. It will also ensure that you get the most important questions answered. Some possible questions?

- ♥ What age group do you typically work with?
- ♥ What is your perspective on preventive care?
- ♥ How do you involve patients in healthcare decisions?

After interviewing each doctor, take your own emotional temperature. Were you comfortable and at ease? Was the doctor? Did he or she take the time to answer all of your questions and answer them clearly? If you feel confident with the physician, your choice is made.

Make an Appointment

Once you have made your choice, it is time to make a medical appointment. This will be the time for a full examination and medical history. The doctor should ask a full slate of questions. He or she will want to know about your family health history and your health history as well as other prevailing influences, such as any smoking or alcohol history, psychiatric conditions, etc. If you have any medical records, make sure to bring them with you or have them sent directly to the doctor's office. Bring any and all medications for the doctor to check. It is important to look for potential side effects or drug interactions.

Finally, revisit the question of communication. A doctor-patient relationship is a two-way street. It is important that you hold up your end of the bargain and communicate as openly and honestly as you want the doctor to do. You should be forming a relationship that will nurture confidence and security, as well as confidentiality and privacy. This leads us to advocacy.

Advocating Your Care

This is an issue near and dear to my heart. Yes, I am a physician, but I have also been a patient, and I have dear family and friends who are patients. As a doctor I understand our strengths. We pursue a career that is demanding and requires dedication and commitment. Our educations test us under with rigorous and crazy schedules. We perform surgeries under the tutelage of skilled and watchful mentors. We are well-prepared for the life and lifestyle we choose.

However, in the end, we are as frail and vulnerable as anyone. We wake up in the morning anxious about the upcoming day, realizing that today may be the day that we are asked to tip the scales of life and death. We wake up in the night with fear because we somehow failed a patient. We rejoice with family and friends as they watch their loved one return to health, sometimes due to our skill, sometimes due to fate or the patient's own grit. We are asked to heal, but we also need healing. We are asked to provide guidance, but we too need guiding. We are trained to keep a psychological perspective in the relationship with our patients, but we all cry when our skills or medicine fail. We might have science, logic, and sometimes even brilliance on our side, but without hope and faith we would be lost.

You Diagnose It

Teresa visited my office after being referred by her family doctor. For nearly four years she had been having palpitations and chest tightness that would radiate to her back. These symptoms would normally come on after walking about a city block and go away with rest.

Upon examining her, I learned that she was fifty-six years old. Her pulse was 80, blood pressure 130/80. When I listened to her heart, there were abnormal sounds, called "clicks." Do you have a possible diagnosis?

Discussion

The presence of the "clicks" while listening to her heart was the real key to diagnosis here. My first suspicion—and I turned out to be correct—was mitral-valve prolapse (MVP). This may sound like a scary diagnosis, but in reality, most patients do very, very well with it and do not require any treatment.

Very few patients with MVP may develop a serious arrhythmia, infective endocarditis, thromboembolus, or progressive disease requiring treatment. In even rarer cases, sudden death is a possibility.

However, in Teresa's case, I felt she did not require any treatment. Her general health was good and her symptoms were minimal. They did not seem to inhibit her daily activities. Teresa's brother had recently been diagnosed with severe coronary artery disease, which required a bypass graft. For this reason, she was nervous about the possibility of more extensive problems and requested a coronary arteriography. This test returned normal coronary arteries and the left ventriculogram showed mild mitral insufficiency. All in all, positive results. Teresa was reassured. She follows up with me once a year for a "check up" but continues to do well and is thriving in her day-to-day life.

The reason I make this point is that, although I believe physicians are honed to the finest point, they can still make mistakes. They have families and bills and worries just like the rest of the world. It is possible for them to make a mistake. Maybe they won't have time to return your call or fully research a question. Maybe they will forget to refill your medication or lose track of an important detail.

Mistakes in the medical profession are very rare considering the volume of patients that each doctor sees. Unfortunately, in our world, any mistake is a dangerous mistake. Heaven forbid you find a doctor that is a "bad apple." Though I have never met one personally, I am sure they exist in the physician population as they do in the population at large. For these reasons, it is important for you to be informed and to advocate your own care. Your doctor is your first and best line of defense in your struggles with an illness, but you are an important backup.

Insurance companies provide another layer of information that needs to be managed. You need to understand your condition and treatment enough to be able to interpret the sometimes cryptic hospital bills and insurance statements.

Obviously, I believe in the power of medicine to heal. I see people healed every day. I see them come into the hospital on death's door and walk out with a smile and a wave. They go on to live long, healthy, productive lives. Medicine can do that, but because we place so much hope in something that is as much art as science, our expectations as patients take on a life of their own. No one but the patient can remove the shroud of mystery that exists between them and their physician.

There are several things you can do to advocate for your care.

- ♥ Communicate honestly with your doctor or doctors. Ask them to be direct with you—and you need to be honest and direct in return.
- ♥ Understand your rights. Every hospital has a patient's bill of rights. It is a good idea to ask for a copy if it is not offered to you. It is your right to refuse any medical treatment or test that you choose. Obviously, if your doctor orders a test or procedure, he or she feels it is in your best interest, but it never hurts to question something that makes you feel uncomfortable.
- ♥ Be informed. Always double-check medication name and doses. Be certain that you understand each medication you are prescribed. If you have a chronic condition, it is best to be as educated as possible about the disease. If you are receiving ongoing treatment, there may be times that you are more knowledgeable about your treatment than some of the nurses or laboratory technicians you might encounter.

All states also have laws that govern patient rights. If the need arises, seek out this information by calling your local ombudsman or health advocacy group. Some of the "rights" that are commonly legislated:

- ♥ Right of access to healthcare and continuity of care
- ♥ Processes for filing complaints
- ♥ Medical disclosure requirements
- ♥ Emergency care rights and procedures
- ♥ Nondiscrimination policies

A Word about Costs and Insurance

Over 44 million Americans are uninsured. This is an astronomical number in view of the fact that medical care is almost completely out of reach without insurance. The costs of medical care have become so high, due to a variety of reasons, that for most people, even those in high-income brackets, insurance is essential. And that is for the day-to-day costs. If a catastrophic illness were to befall you, insurance becomes an absolute lifeline.

Having good coverage through an employer is not a fail-safe, either. Co-payments and premiums are skyrocketing while employers attempt to shift more responsibility for costs onto their employees. There is a new trend toward the creation of personal-health accounts. These are pools of money that are available to pay for medical expenses, but the where and how is totally at the discretion of the employee. The theory is that if the employees decide how and when to spend their limited dollars, they will use the money more judiciously and therefore keep costs down. The critics of the plan argue that employees will most often be making critical decisions when they are ill and that the overall amount available is considerably less than with the traditional indemnity plans.

Spending for healthcare increased nearly seven percent in 2000, and insurance premiums for employers went up an average of eleven percent in 2001, with no end in sight. Increasing costs for hospital services and prescription drugs are the primary driving factor for these increases. Employees are increasingly paying for these increases as well. Employers are passing along 50-80% of these increases to their employees.

What can you do to best protect yourself? Here are some recommendations.

- ♥ Write healthcare costs into your budget. Treat these costs as given and necessary. Leave additional money for unexpected increases in co-payments or a sudden illness.
- ♥ Don't be tempted to go without. Even if you never develop a serious illness or chronic condition, insurance pays for itself merely by providing preventive care.
- ♥ Be wary of personal health accounts if they are offered by your employer. They are not a good option if you have a chronic illness, and the deductibles can be exceptionally high.
- ♥ When you are ill, the last thing anyone wants to worry about is how to pay for the care. At that time, the single most important thing is getting the care that you desperately need. Nothing else matters.

I hope the time never comes for you, but as my mother is fond of saying, "Plan for the worst and hope for the best." None of us want to believe that we will fall ill and need extended care, but the statistics tell us otherwise. If you have questions about insurance and finances, seek out a trustworthy financial counselor rather than an insurance agent. Deal with an accountant or financial advisor to work out costs and budgeting, and you will have a good base to work from when negotiating with an insurance agent or employer. A good financial advisor can tell you where your money is best spent, how much to hold in reserve or savings, and how much you can reasonably afford to put toward healthcare costs. This will help when making many financial decisions regarding healthcare.

As a physician who struggles with insurance and payment issues everyday, I wish that we had a utopian society with a perfect system. However, we have what we have, and we work through it in the best way we can while waiting for the healthcare and insurance reform that is on the horizon.

As a consumer, know your rights, know your finances, and know your limits. Remember that your physicians are on your team, but never abrogate your rights to speak for yourself and to question decisions where necessary. Build a solid working relationship with your healthcare team, and it will be there to serve you when you need it most.

CHAPTER 7

Be Good to Your Heart: Finding Balance

Finding Balance

I should be the last one to include a discussion about balance in a book. I have never been a particularly patient person, and I am certainly a "perfectionist." I have always been driven to do more and to do it faster and better than I have before. I feel that I owe my patients no less than this commitment. I take my work so seriously that it often precludes other things in life that are important as well. You may have heard stories about medical school and internship. Surgeons working on less than two hours of sleep at a time or interns pulling shifts for 48-72 straight hours. I wish I could say these stories were exaggerated. For better or worse, physicians are trained by trial of fire. The thought is, if they can work under these arduous circumstances, they can be trusted to make difficult decisions on a daily basis.

Unfortunately, I haven't cornered the market on perfectionism, stress, or imbalance. I see the symptoms of these traits walk through the door of my clinic everyday. I see hearts torn completely apart by their own strength and passion. What requires more commitment than being a mother? Who has more ambition than a woman bucking the odds to get ahead at work? Where can you find more passion than a young woman searching for love or falling in love? I don't mean, in any way, to say that women work only by emotion, but to their favor, they do not shy from them. In the end, this works to their benefit and to their detriment.

I believe—and this is confirmed by my years of caring for hearts—that the best and perhaps the only way to ensure a healthy heart is to achieve emotional well being and balance in life. If, as human beings, we were able to strike a perfect unison in diet, movement, and spirit, our bodies would hang in a sort of suspended animation in terms of disease and aging. Of course, this perfection is not to be found in our corporeal existence.

Even though we run the risk of "stressing" as we add the pressure to our lives of trying to achieve "balance," it is a pressure that we must acknowledge. The road to health takes us across that bridge, and there is no other path.

We are going to look at diet, movement, and spirit individually and as a triad. They exist separately and in concert. For example, diets nourish or degrade our bodies, the course often determined by emotional pressures. The amount of movement in our daily lives is determined not only by our physical reserves but our mental state as well. Our ability to devote time to spiritual matters is often helped or hindered by physical health and emotional states. We will look at the dysfunctions that can arise in these three areas, but more importantly, we will talk about what good health "looks like." We have spent much of the book discussing diseases and their various states. It is now time to turn our attention to health. I hope to give you a solid picture of what it might look like to have balanced health (though there are infinite presentations) in order to give you a positive focus. The early chapters of this book have provided the technical and scientific information you need to be an informed patient. After this chapter, you will have images drawn at an emotional and spiritual level as well. It is my hope you will gain a holistic view of your health, tempered with the latest in medicine, so that you will have all of the tools at your disposal to ensure that your heart remains as healthy as possible.

Diet

Diets are killing people, not only in America but the world over. The increased consumption of processed foods and refined sugars is taking its toll on waistlines as well as lives. Beyond the physical toll, we need to deal with the reality of the emotional toll. Women, more than ever, are plagued with "ideal" body images portrayed in popular culture. They are left to fend for themselves in building a healthy sense of self-image. Women are also under more stress than ever before. They are holding jobs, nurturing children, running households, and caring for husbands—and losing themselves in the process. We don't need a psychiatrist to tell us that many women retreat to "comfort" food as a way of nourishing themselves and recuperating from the intense pressure they face in day-to-day life.

A dear friend of mine called me to relate her fears about her sister. It seemed that her sister, who was thirty-one at the time, had developed anorexia and bulimia. She was eating only granola and non-fat yogurt. If she did manage to eat something outside of those boundaries, she would binge and then throw it all up.

My friend wanted to know if her sister was truly anorexic. I had to admit to my ignorance of eating disorders. I know only what I learned in a few semesters of psychology in school.

In order to feel helpful, I asked a few doctor-like questions. How old was she? When did this start? What was her health like currently? What surfaced was an interesting portrait of a strong woman who seemed to be crumpling beneath the weight of incredible stress. In the span of one year, she had suffered two miscarriages and the loss of a beloved horse she had owned for more than twenty years. Her children were growing and presenting new stresses, and her work was demanding. I was told that she was a labor-and-delivery nurse who had come into contact with HIV helping a mother to pump breast milk. The original tests were false positives, and she suffered for months believing she had contracted this terrifying disease. She journeyed through the entire spectrum of life and death within a short period of time and had turned all of her grief and pain inward; in the end it manifested as anorexia.

This was more than enough uncertainty, fear, and loss for a lifetime, let alone a short year. I struggled with myself, the heroic doctor against the faulty human. I had no basis from which to understand this woman, nor did I have any basis from which to psychoanalyze her, but the doctor in me rose to meet the challenge. My friend was fearful and her sister was in pain and killing herself, albeit slowly. Was there nothing I could offer?

In the end, the answer surprised me. I wanted to get in there with my scalpel and excise the demons taking over this woman's life. I imagined, much like an appendix, there was some useless piece of anatomy I could remove that would take away her sorrow, but the battle being waged inside of her heart was on an intimate level. Who was I to pierce the shroud of intimacy under the pretense of "helping" her?

As a physician, I know about the physicality of a woman's heart. I know she was inflicting damage with the diet and vomiting. The retching would damage the heart muscles and reverse the muscles in her esophagus. The acid in the reflux would erode the lining of her throat and eat the enamel of her teeth. The vomiting would disturb the balance of electrolytes in her system, leading to damage in other organs as well. In spite of my knowledge and education, the best I could offer was friendship.

The Flip Side

Of course, this young woman is an extreme case. Anorexia and bulimia occur in only about 5% of the population, but of this five percent, 90% are females. On the other side, nearly 59% of the total population is either overweight or obese. This statistic alone accounts for the gigantic diet industry and demonstrates the day-to-day struggle that over half the population faces, the struggle to maintain a healthy body weight. This call prompted me to examine the concept of food on a different level. Why do some people respond to stress or a need for comfort by overeating or eating poorly while others strip themselves of the right to eat anything at all?

Obviously, this question won't be answered in this book. It is not the proper forum, nor do I possess expertise on the subject. However, I would like you to consider this question as you read the rest of this chapter. Do you fall into one of these extreme groups? If so, how did food come to mean more than sustenance for you?

If you are in the 50% of the population that is not overweight, are you making the appropriate food choices or do you choose your meals based on emotional issues as well? Emotional eating is not the domain of the anorexic or obese. We all fall into the habit at one time or another.

Shopping Tips

Healthy diet starts with good shopping habits. If you don't have the extra sugar in the house, you can't eat it. If you buy red meat only a few times a month, it won't sit in the freezer tempting you. Here are some shopping tips you can use to help you with the transition to better nutrition.

- Buy as many fresh foods as possible. Avoid the processed and frozen-food aisles. Work your way around the edge of the outside aisles of the store and avoid the inner aisles, where the refined foods are usually kept.
- Check food labels for hidden sugars or sodium.
- Have a plan. Work out a week's worth of meals and make a list accordingly. If it's not on the list, don't buy it!
- Take your time when you're shopping, and never, ever shop when you are hungry!

I raise this issue because it is ground zero for the viral-like spread of obesity in our population. It would be pointless to discuss healthy diet from a physical standpoint alone when the majority of us need guidance from an emotional perspective as well.

The Fads

As mentioned earlier, diet is an important contributor to a healthy heart. I spend a large percentage of my office time consulting with my patients about their diet. It is a controllable factor. We don't have dominance over our genetic history, but we can manage our diet. Unfortunately, the diet industry does little to help me in this regard. Every six weeks, a new diet plan sweeps across the nation. Commonly and tragically, the focus is typically on weight and not on health.

Can I blame the majority for believing in these plans? No. They all have basic tenets that make sense. The problem occurs when the diets are too one-sided or extreme. Take the infamous grapefruit diet as an example. Is grapefruit good for you? Can it do the things they said it could? The answer to these questions is yes, it can, and it does. That does not mean that one should eat a diet consisting entirely of grapefruit. It seems almost ridiculous now that such a thing could have been asserted.

Helpful Supplements

There are many nutrients and supplements that are beneficial to your heart. Here are a few to consider.

- ♥ **Folic Acid**: Recommended dose is 400 micrograms a day. Reduces heart disease by 31%. Decreases homocysteine levels in the blood. Can be found in orange juice, kidney beans, broccoli, and spinach. Folic acid is especially good for pregnant moms. It has been found to decrease the incidence of spina bifida in newborns.
- ♥ **Vitamin B6**: Recommend 3 mg per day. Lowers the risk of heart disease by 33%. Also lowers homocysteine levels in the blood. Eat bananas, avocados, lean chicken, brown rice, and oats for this nutrient.
- ♥ **Vitamin E**: 400 IU/day. Reduces incidence of heart disease by 40%. Reduces incidence of second heart attack by 77%. You can find vitamin E in vegetable oils, nuts, and wheat germ.
- ♥ **Omega-3**: This is a valuable oil found mainly in fatty fish. Reduces heart spasms and platelet clumping, as well as reducing the risk of heart attack by 50% to 70%.
- ♥ **Lycopene**: This nutrient is known to prevent heart disease and cancer. It is found in tomatoes, especially those that are cooked. It is best to use a bit of olive oil in addition because it helps to aid absorption.
- ♥ **Flavanoid**: This is a blood-thinning agent. It can be found in grapes, apples, onions, and tea. Grape juice twice a day reduces clotting by 60%.

How about the plans that offer quick weight loss, as in the diets that promise you will lose 10 pounds in a week? Do they work? Usually. Are they healthy? Absolutely not. Is the weight loss permanent? Almost never. Metabolically, it is impossible for your body to keep up with the rapid changes in diet and exercise that these plans espouse. Just when the body slows down its metabolism to accommodate the fewer calories, the dieter has reached their goal or is weakening in their resolve and increases their caloric intake. What happens? The body is not able to use the calories fast enough and the weight is gained back, and then some. This becomes a never-ending loop—the yo-yo diet that we have come to fear.

The Magic Bullet

In science and medicine, researchers are always looking for the magic bullet. They search for a protein that will bind to the surface of a cell and destroy a cancer. They look for an enzyme that will metabolize in such a way as to reduce cholesterol. Their quests are noble, and thankfully, many breakthroughs have been achieved as of late. Great strides are being made in the understanding of the human body, disease processes, and other physiological phenomena.

When it comes to diet, however, science is still woefully inadequate. We have an understanding of the metabolic processes. We know the basics of the digestive system and its work. We have a general idea about what constitutes healthy nutrition in terms of vitamins, minerals, proteins, fats, and sugars.

There have been great amounts of research done in these areas, but we still have a lot to learn. Because the human body can vary greatly from individual to individual with respect to fat storage, propensity towards a body type, conversion of cholesterols, etc., it is difficult to define a diet that will work for everyone. When you throw in considerations of temperament, tastes, and emotions, the subject becomes complicated even further.

Normal Food or Diet Food

In response to some of this confusion, a study called the Lyon Diet Heart Study was performed. Anecdotally, researchers knew that certain areas of the Mediterranean had the lowest recorded rates of chronic disease and the highest life expectancies. Diet was revealed as a causative factor in this good fortune. In 1999, the final report of the Lyon study revealed that the Mediterranean diet reduced the chances of a second heart attack or sudden death by about 70%. This is an astonishing number! The researchers felt that a big part of the diet's success was related to the high amounts of a particular type of omega-3 fatty acid commonly found in soybeans, canola oils, and fish.

A typical resident of the Mediterranean area will eat red meat only a few times a month; sweets, eggs, poultry, and fish a few times a week; and cheese or yogurt, olive oil, fruits, beans, legumes, nuts, and vegetables daily, in addition to breads, rice, pasta, and other starches.

For many years, the low-fat/high-carbohydrate diet was touted as the best for your heart. Many cardiologists followed this line of thinking. The point was to decrease the intake of bad fats as much as possible. This was offset with carbohydrates, which were thought to burn quickly and provide efficient energy. As it turns out, this thinking was off the mark. The extra calories from refined carbohydrates (breads, bagels, pastas, waffles, sweets) are stored as fat. Also, the sugar content of these foods causes "insulin resistance" within the body. The body is simply not able to utilize all of the sugars being introduced into the bloodstream.

The other problem that arises with a low-fat diet is a lack of necessary fats, such as the healthy fatty acids provided by a Mediterranean diet. Olive oil in moderation provides key fatty acids that are needed to raise the "good" cholesterol in your bloodstream. The same is true of fish and other foods common in this area.

With all of that said, the Mediterranean diet isn't really a "diet." After all, for thousands of people, it is their normal, natural choice, not something they force upon themselves to attain health or ideal weight. People in these regions have eaten similar foods for centuries.

I have a patient who was very successful in maintaining a healthy diet based on the Mediterranean style of eating. I asked her how she managed to do it without ever complaining to me once.

"Doctor," she said, "my husband took me on a trip once to Italy. The people, the places, the smells, the foods—they are all imprinted on my mind. It was the best three weeks of my entire life. When I think I would rather eat a piece of cake than a piece of fruit, I just think of the wonderful blue sea near Capri. I feel the warm air and taste the flavor of fresh-from-the-field grapes. What is there to complain about?"

This patient had found a unique but remarkable way to make associations with healthy food choices that made her feel good rather than bad. She had also found a way to "normalize" the foods she was eating, rather than thinking in terms of "dieting." I have to admit, I use her technique frequently when I find myself tempted by a donut rather than fresh strawberries.

The Mediterranean Way

So, what exactly is the Mediterranean way of eating, and why should you adopt it?

First of all, I recommend making diet changes slowly. You are looking to establish a habit that will last for the whole of your life. You stand a better chance of making the emotional adjustment if you make the changes slowly and incorporate them fully into your life.

Secondly, I am not going to put forth a specific diet. There are many excellent books on the subject, and we have listed them in the Resources section of the appendix. If you would like detailed information or direction, any one of these books would be helpful. I would, however, like to offer some suggestions for changes in direction. These are subtle, easy-to-make corrections that you can incorporate into your lifestyle.

- Limit your intake of any type of refined or processed foods. This is true for commercial cereals, breads, and pastries, as well as sweets containing large amounts of refined sugar. The motto of "everything in moderation" is especially true when making food choices.
- Try to get in as many fresh fruits and vegetables as you possibly can in a day, particularly leafy greens, broccoli, brussel sprouts, and any kind of fruit. Bear in mind that bananas, grapes, and melons contain more sugar than fruits like cherries, peaches, pears, and apples.
- Include onions, garlic, and herbs in your cooking. They each have unique chemical properties that combat cholesterol and assist the immune system.
- Avoid foods with hydrogenated oils. If you avoid processed foods such as cakes, chips, and crackers, you will be avoiding these oils.
- Take your dairy in the form of cheese and yogurt and avoid milk. Milk has a higher sugar content and contributes more readily to insulin resistance.
- Minimize the consumption of red meat (maybe only a few times a month) and increase your intake of fatty fish.
- Snack on nuts and seeds. Flaxseed oil is a great source of omega-3 fatty acids. It can be bought in the refrigerated section of most health food departments. It is easy to mix into a salad or vegetables. Keep in mind not to use it in cooking, however. If it is heated, the oil can become carcinogenic.
- Watch out for hidden sources of sugar, such as processed fruit juices. Be conscious of your salt intake, particularly if you use canned vegetables—they are typically high in sodium.

The Mediterranean area is famous for its wine consumption, and there is some evidence that drinking one glass of wine a day aids digestion, decreases cholesterol levels, and provides other benefits. The key here is moderation. Women should drink only one glass of wine a day, where men might be allowed two. If you don't already drink, don't start. You can achieve the same benefit by eating fresh grapes or drinking grape juice.

Eating For Your Heart

Eating and "not eating" can both be addictions. There is a clear emotional underpinning to the way we use food in our lives.

Additionally, science is still learning about physiology and nutrition. A very recent study done by Dr. Lars Skodstan in Sweden found that the Mediterranean diet reduced the pain and improved the physical functioning of people with rheumatoid arthritis. He believes there is a connection between this type of arthritis and heart disease. Clearly there is a connection to diet. This style of eating has also been associated with a decreased risk of cancer, as well as osteoporosis, and there is still much more to discover about the benefits of healthy foods.

Connecting

Diets, dieting, and other food-related obsessions have become a central part of modern society. Every few days another study comes out telling us what or what not to eat. In the end, it is very simple: everything in moderation. The complications arise when we find that we have connected food sustenance with dysfunctional emo-

Time Out

A patient of mine was in for a visit and brought along her three-year-old son. He was an animated child—very intelligent and into everything in the office. She definitely had her hands full parenting this young man. She wanted to encourage his curiosity and intellect without allowing him to completely disrupt the surrounding environment. He was fascinated with the instruments and their uses and picked up all the tidbits of information that I was dispensing. I was impressed with how fast he grasped some pretty difficult concepts and fancied myself a mentor to a young protégé. Just when I was feeling full of myself and about to go into a lecture about the nobility of the medical profession, he picked up a stethoscope. I watched him anxiously to see if he would remember its use, as I had carefully explained it just a few moments ago. Instead he spoke into the instrument,

"Welcome to McDonald's. May I take your order?" So much for MY ego.

tional nurturing. The diet proponents would have a much easier time of getting their diets to work if they would address the emotional issues. Then again, if the emotional issues were properly dealt with, a diet would not be necessary.

The point is to eat right for your body, mind, and heart. It can be painful to strip down your conception of food and change your mindset from "diet" to "health." I hope the next sections on movement and spirituality will give you some ideas that will make the transition easier.

The Lost Art: Herbal Supplements

In early days we were close to nature. The good earth, the blue sky, the flying of geese, and the changing winds...we lived by God's hand through nature.
—Unknown Speaker, Addressing the National Congress of American Indians

Once the domain of shamans (tribal religious leaders) and folklore-inspired healers, herbs have made the jump into mainstream culture. We know the ancient Sumerians, nearly 5000 years ago, were using laurel, caraway, and thyme for medicinal purposes. After hundreds of years of trial-and-error experimentation, the Chinese Herb Book, written in 2700 B.C., documented 365 medicinal plants and their uses, including *ma-huang*. Ma-huang, as we will learn later, is the shrub that is used to produce ephedrine. As the seventeenth century approached, there was a slow erosion of the use of plants as medicine. Soon thereafter, chemical drugs were introduced, followed by the rapid development of chemistry and other physical sciences.

We go in search of "natural" remedies when science disappoints us. Self-medication in the form of herbs and other supplements continues to rise in popularity, in spite of rapid advances in conventional medicine. In a recent study, 40% of the population reported herb use, with the majority of that percentage being women (Klepser 2000). As one would expect, most of these people believe that these herbal remedies benefit them in some way or other. What surprises me about this study, however, is these same people believe their physicians view herbal supplements as being beneficial as well. They assume conventional medicine shares their perspective on alternative therapies. Poll a handful of doctors and you will find this is simply not true, and for good reason.

Hidden Dangers

Many, many herbs have pharmacokinetic properties. They can be used to remedy constipation, elevate mood, reduce blood sugar, or assist with weight loss. Most of them have scientifically valid uses. However, as with pharmaceutical drugs, they are not all harmless. They have powerful effects and need to be handled with care. We often have the false assumption that anything natural is harmless. I would, in fact, postulate the opposite. Nature is very powerful and should be handled with care. Ancient herbal remedies formed the basis for many of our current medicines. They have potent chemical properties that can inflict damage or illness if not used correctly.

We have lost the traditional knowledge about herbs and healing. The onset of scientific research and the use of chemicals led us away from the natural world and into a chemistry lab. True, modern drugs and drug research had their start in the plant world, but we are now removed from the original forms as they were known thousands of years ago. As humans, we have the intuitive sense that there is healing in these plants, and we are correct. However, in times gone by, healing (even with herbs) was done by a practitioner of the art who understood the uses of each plant. It would have been unthinkable for an "average" person to medicate him or herself. Such things were left to the religious leaders or healers.

The FDA offers little assistance in regulating these drugs. Herbs and other supplements which are classified as weight loss substances are not regulated in the manner that pharmaceutical drugs have been. Just because it is carried on the market does not mean that it has been safety-tested or studied. It does not mean that the claims made about its healing properties have been scientifically proven.

With respect to heart disease, we do know of many herbs that can be helpful, but there are more that are dangerous and interact negatively with cardiac medications. Some do both. Let's take a look at a few of the more widely-used herbs.

Table 7.1

Common Medicinal Herbs

Name	Effects, Uses and Toxicities	Interactions
Alfalfa	May aggravate lupus and other auto-immune diseases.	
Aloe	Potent laxative. Not to be used internally by pregnant women, children, or the elderly.	
Angelica	Excess dosage can negatively affect blood pressure, heart rate, and respiration. Absolutely not to be used during pregnancy or if you are experiencing a heavy cycle.	
Borage Seed Oil	Long-term intake may cause toxicity.	
Cascara	Useful mild laxative but not for use during pregnancy or while nursing.	
Chamomile	Causes vessels to dilate.	Warfarin
Echinacea	Boosts immunity. May cause allergic reactions. Impairs immune-suppressive drugs. Can cause immune suppression when taken long-term. May impair wound healing.	Discontinue far in advance of surgery.
Ephedra	Increases heart rate and blood pressure. Increased risk of heart attack, arrhythmia, stroke, kidney stones, and interactions with other drugs. Women particularly demonstrate increased risk of stroke. Used for weight loss, but risks outweigh benefits.	Discontinue prior to surgery. *** FDA Ban from Market ***
Feverfew	Causes vessels to dilate. Useful for migraines. Inhibits clotting and release of serotonin.	Warfarin and anticoagulants
Garlic	Inhibits clotting.	Warfarin. Discontinue 7 days before surgery.
Ginger	Associated with prolonged bleeding time.	Warfarin
Ginkgo	Safe for circulatory disturbances, claudication, memory impairment.	Aspirin, NSAIDs, warfarin, heparin. Discontinue 36 hours before surgery.
Ginseng	Falsely elevated digoxin levels, increases blood pressure, insomnia, vomiting, headache, nose bleeds, nervousness. Lowers blood glucose.	Warfarin, phenelzine. Discontinue 7 days before surgery.
Gossypol	Kidney loss of potassium.	Hydrochlorothiazide, furosemide, digoxin.
Kava	Sedative. Decreases anxiety. Risks of addiction, tolerance, and withdrawal unknown.	May increase sedative effects of anesthesia. Discontinue 5 days before surgery.

Table 7.1

Common Medicinal Herbs, continued

Name	Effects, Uses and Toxicities	Interactions
Kelp	Hyperthyroidism. Atrial fibrillation in some people.	Amiodarone.
Licorice	Associated with loss of potassium and hypokalemia.	Digoxin, spironolactone.
St. John's Wort	Sedative. Decreases anxiety. Anti-depressant effect. Avoid tyramine-containing foods such as red wine, cheese, yeast, and pickled herring. Absolutely not for use during pregnancy or with other anti-depressant medications.	Alters metabolism of other drugs. Discontinue 5 days before surgery.
Valerian Root	Sedative. May increase effects of other sedatives. Long-term use could increase the amount of anesthesia needed during surgery. Withdrawal symptoms resemble Valium addiction.	Taper dose before surgery. Treat withdrawal symptoms with benzodiazepines.

If you are interested in using herbs as a part of your health routine, I highly recommend working with your physician. Let them know what you are interested in taking and ask for their perspective. It is vital that you cross-check any medications you may be taking to make sure that they will not interact. I encourage all of my patients to be active participants in their own healthcare. I also encourage them to open a dialogue with me so that I can help them work through questions and concerns. In the end, if a patient makes the decision to continue with a supplement against my advice, we agree to disagree; The patient is in charge.

In the instance of pregnancy or nursing, I strongly advise against the use of herbal remedies. Most are transmittable through the placenta and may affect an unborn child. There simply has not been enough scientific research done showing that supplements do not adversely affect pregnancy. Please, please be certain to check with your obstetrician if you intend to take any herbal remedies, including herbal tea.

Finally, with respect specifically to heart health, there is no magic cure for high cholesterol, obesity, or high blood pressure. The best cure is to eat intelligently and to get an appropriate amount of exercise. Keep an eye on your stress levels and be sure to get enough rest.

Modern science is truly miraculous, but there are important pieces missing that can never be put in place. In our era of specialization, it would not be likely to have one person birth you and care for you from the beginning of your life near to the end, as a tribal elder might have. In light of this, it is no surprise we seek out an older wisdom, something more connected to the earth. We have genetic memories of life in a village, a life dependent upon other humans and buoyed by the natural world. For better or worse, we live in a different time.

Movement

Why do strong arms fatigue themselves with frivolous dumbbells? To dig a vineyard is worthier exercise for men.
—Marcus Valerius Martialis

Let me start this section of the chapter with some good news: I do NOT believe in exercise. I think exercise is a formal construct that only serves to augment our guilt when it comes to taking care of our bodies. Unless you are an athlete with specific goals in mind, a formal exercise program is simply not necessary for your heart health.

As you might expect, there is a flip side to this bit of news. You do not have to exercise, but you do have to move. Movement, in and of itself, is what our bodies were made for. From the beginning of our creation (whatever form that takes for you), we have evolved to move. The very nature of our two-legged, upright walking structure is designed to get us from one place to another as quickly as possible. As I mentioned previously, if you stand still in one place too long, blood pools up in your legs and this can cause you to faint. The heart, as powerful as it is, still needs the muscles and movement of the body to assist it in its work.

Heart disease, to the extent that we know it now, is a relatively recent phenomenon. There are many reasons for this, but one important concept is that we are MOVING less. Until the recent technology age, the majority of occupations required some type of physical exertion. Daily life revolved around physical labor. Now, we don't even have to work for our food; simply roll up to the drive-thru window and hand over some cash. Eating doesn't even require the exertion of going to the refrigerator or standing over the stove while a meal is cooking. For us, food comes easy, prepackaged, precooked, ready to go. This is a far cry from the days of hunting and gathering, when the process of obtaining food was strenuous and difficult.

I believe the best way to attain appropriate amounts of movement is to live an active life. By this, I don't mean working out at the gym three times a week until you can bench press 250 pounds. Goals, in this instance, are just not helpful. Heart healthy movement is not about losing weight, running until you drop, or trying to keep up with the young girl on the treadmill next to you. Who needs all that aggravation? Healthy movement should be a way of life, an integrated part of your lifestyle, not just something you schedule in your day planner and might or might not get to. Exercise plans do come in handy if your life is so harried that you absolutely have to schedule time to exercise, but this is not my recommended course. I ask you to temporarily put aside the stumbling blocks that keep you from feeling you can lead an active life. Put them aside just long enough to read the balance of this chapter. It is my hope, when we are done, that you will have a clear vision of why you DESERVE to move.

Why?

Movement is not a punishment. It is not something to be dreaded or feared. It is a natural function of our physical being. We are designed to move. Can you remember back to the time of your childhood? Picture a warm spring day. What was your favorite activity outside? Can you recall riding your bike with the wind blowing your hair back and feeling so free that nothing could stop you? Do you have memories of running races with you friends, maybe never winning but reveling in the effort? Maybe your joy was feeling warm water slide past as you swam from one edge of the pool to the other. If you were a bit strange, as I was, you may have found it entertaining to see how far you could swim while holding your breath, pushing it just to the point of blacking out. Children love these feelings of freedom. They take happiness and pride in their physicality. They push the limits of their physical endurance when given a chance. They are constantly testing their boundaries, calling on inner strength as well as physical strength. Somewhere in the process of growing up, we lose these freedoms. I can't say for certain whether they are taken away or whether we give them up, but it is certain that we do lose them.

How can we regain that sense of wildness and spirit that inspired us as children? Well, as adults, our logic often gets in the way, so let's give the brain something to work with first.

We all know that exercise is "good for us," but do you know why? Do you know exactly what it does for your body? Here are some specific benefits:

- ♥ Decreased percentage of body fat
- ♥ Increased muscle size, tone, and definition
- ♥ Increased strength and endurance
- ♥ Reduce "bad" cholesterol and increased "good" cholesterol
- ♥ Improved resting blood pressure and metabolic rate
- ♥ Increased insulin sensitivity

Since activity improves your strength and endurance, it also leads to an increased sense of confidence. You no longer have to feel nervous about a flight of stairs or the strain of carrying heavy groceries home. You know you have the strength to change a tire or bike the last few miles with your child. As they credit-card commercial says: Cost of bike: $300. Two hours biking with your son: Priceless. There is simply no way to measure the mental and emotional benefits of feeling fit and healthy. My mother used to demonstrate considerable stamina every fall, when she would work at putting food up for the winter. She would be on her feet from dawn until well past dark. Some people will say that health is not everything, and strangely enough I agree. I think a strong spirit and a sense of humanity outweigh physical health, but feeling strong physically impacts our capacity to feel strong mentally and emotionally as well.

How, When, and Where?

Now that we have looked at some of the whys, let's look at the how, when, and where. I can sum this up very simply: however, whenever, wherever. As I said before, movement is a way of life. You must incorporate it into your lifestyle if you want to give your heart its best chances. Let's look at an extreme case.

I have a friend who is a triathlete. She lives the epitome of a scheduled and measured lifestyle. She works 40-60 hours a week, and every minute of her time outside of work is devoted to her preparations for triathlon. She weighs and measures everything she eats, mostly to make sure she is getting enough to eat. She takes in excess of 5,000 calories a day just to break even with her expenditures. She is up at 5:00 A.M. to go swimming and is out on the streets running or biking the second she leaves work. On the weekends she spends six to eight hours each day running or biking. Family priorities are not an issue because she is not married and doesn't have children.

Stay on the Couch!

There is one time I advocate staying on the couch rather than heading out for a walk. Your risk of heart attack is four times greater within two hours of eating an unusually heavy meal. According to a study presented at the American Heart Association's Scientific Sessions in 2000, overeating itself may increase the risk of heart attacks. Having a big meal can adversely affect the heart by increasing the heart rate, blood pressure, and oxygen requirements. All of these factors cause the heart to work harder at its job, by:

- Increasing insulin, which reduces the relaxation of the coronary arteries
- High blood pressure, which may cause the cholesterol deposits to break away from the vessel wall, creating a clot that will eventually block a blood vessel
- Exercise, which reduces the amount of adrenaline in your system, which lowers your pulse rate. It can also increase the amount of endorphins, which elevate mood and feelings of well being. If I have a patient come in that is suffering from depression, my first recommendation is that she increase her activity levels. We work out specific ways that she can get more activity, even strenuous activity. In the majority of my patients, exercise alone has been enough treatment for their depression. I am not suggesting it is enough in all cases, but it is a place to start.

Therefore, if you indulge in a big holiday meal, save the game of touch football for later. Light activity, if you are used to exertion, is not a problem, but don't exert yourself past what you would normally consider a gentle workout.

She may be everything I advocate against in terms of methods, but I can't argue with the results. For her, triathlon is who she is. It is a part of her. She thrives on the competition and challenge and would wither without it. Fortunately for her, she has chosen a "habit" that is healthy. There may be a few of you who have chosen the same route. If you are a woman with a strong competitive drive, a scheduled program may work to your benefit. In fact, it might be a necessity if you are to come out ahead of your competitors. However, if you find it hard to make time to stop and catch your breath, let's consider a different approach, an approach based more on philosophy.

Let's take a look at an average day in the life of Jessica, a young woman who has two children and works a nine-to-five job.

- ♥ 6:00 A.M. Out of bed, shower, dress.
- ♥ 6:45 A.M. Make breakfast and lunches.

- ♥ 7:15 A.M. See kids to school bus, commute to work.
- ♥ 8:00 A.M. Arrive at work. Majority of the day spent at desk with computer work. Take-out lunch at desk.
- ♥ 5:00 P.M. Pick up kids at after-school care. Commute home.
- ♥ 5:30 P.M. Make and eat dinner.
- ♥ 6:15 P.M. Dishes.
- ♥ 6:30 P.M. Help kids with homework.
- ♥ 7:30 P.M. Take kids to karate class. Read a book while waiting.
- ♥ 8:30 P.M. Back home and get the children into bed.
- ♥ 9:00 P.M. Catch up on housework.
- ♥ 10:00 P.M. Get into bed for the night.

Okay, okay, before you shoot me down, I know this is a LIGHT schedule in a perfect world. After all, who ever gets a complete eight hours of sleep a night? I am just trying to give an average picture here. Let's take this same schedule and total up the amount of light-to-moderate exercise Jessica got during this day. Her grand total of light exercise for the day would be about an hour, the time she spent cleaning the house in the evening. At no other time during her day was her heart rate likely to be above baseline, if we factor out stress responses. Physically, she did not tax her body at all, until it came to the housework, and even then it would depend on whether she was actively scrubbing floors or just picking up clutter.

Here is how I might suggest Jessica structure her day to obtain a healthy amount of exercise. Again, please remember, these are just suggestions. Not everyone could incorporate all of these changes. They are just food for thought.

- ♥ 5:45 A.M. Get out of bed, 15-minute walk, shower, dress.
- ♥ 6:45 A.M. Make breakfast and lunches.
- ♥ 7:15 A.M. See kids to school bus, ride bike or walk to work.
- ♥ 8:00 A.M. Arrive at work. Spend 2 hours at desk. Take a 15-minute break for a short walk. Spend another 2 hours working.
- ♥ 12:00 P.M. Either take an hour-long walk and eat a healthy lunch at desk or a 15-minute walk each way to a nearby restaurant for lunch.
- ♥ 1:00 P.M. Work 4 hours at desk with a 15-minute walking break halfway through.
- ♥ 5:00 P.M. Pick up kids at after-school care. Ride bikes or walk home.
- ♥ 5:30 P.M. Make and eat dinner. Relax with some quiet music or talking with kids about their day.

- ♥ 6:15 P.M. Do the dishes. Time to liven things up with some energetic music. Dance a little while doing dishes. The kids will LOVE it. (If they are teenagers, they will be VERY embarrassed, which is almost as good.)
- ♥ 6:30 P.M. Help kids with homework.
- ♥ 7:30 P.M. Take kids to karate class. Join class or spend time in your own activity of choice.
- ♥ 8:30 P.M. Go back home and get the children into bed.
- ♥ 9:00 P.M. Catch up on housework, make sure to include vigorous work, such as vacuuming or washing windows.
- ♥ 10:00 P.M. Get into bed for the night.

Again, this is a perfect schedule in a perfect world, but with a few minor changes, we have managed to squeeze in nearly four hours of activity. This is EIGHT times the recommended half an hour daily. Some of the work is light, but some of it is sufficiently vigorous to increase heart rate. All of it is beneficial to your health and your heart.

I hesitated to present an example like this because there are too many "yes, buts…" that can be thrown up as blockades. The only point I am trying to make is that if you LOOK for ways to incorporate activity into your day, you will find them. Jessica never needs to set foot inside a gym or an aerobics class if she doesn't want to. Of course, she may decide that she enjoys the company of the other women or that she likes the relaxation of the treadmill, but it is not a necessity. There are plenty of other ways for her to "sneak in" her workouts.

It is not necessary to make your heart pound in your chest to realize a good workout. In fact, even elite athletes rarely exert themselves to this point. They carefully build up a base of stamina and endurance and religiously watch their heart rates to keep them in their target zone. For the average person looking to achieve a healthier heart, it is only necessary to get your heart rate to a place where you feel you are "working" but are still able to talk. If you really want a specific heart rate number, you can easily determine your heart rate zone. Here is the formula:

> 220-(Your age) x 70%. This is the low end of the range.
> 220-(Your age) x 85%. This is the high end of the range.

For example, if you are 40 years old, your target range would be 126 to 153. Walking at a reasonable pace for about 5 minutes should easily get your heart into this range. Don't believe me? Try it out. While walking, periodically take your pulse. You can count the beats for fifteen seconds and multiply by four to get an approximate heart rate. If your heart rate is too low, pick up the pace a bit. If it is too fast, definitely slow down.

I have a patient who says she gets her heart rate from 70 to 125 just by sprinting to the backyard when one of her children screams. A few of those sprints everyday and you are nearly a quarter of the way to the recommended half hour of daily exercise.

I would like to add one recommendation here. Especially for women, aerobic exercise is not enough. It is very important that you include some sort of weight-bearing exercise as well. This could be in the traditional form of lifting weights, or you might have more ingenious methods, such as shoveling in the garden or even playing tennis. Studies have shown us that weight-bearing exercise reduces the risk of osteoporosis by stressing the bones and forcing them to work harder at their jobs. Of course, you will achieve the expected results of increased muscle strength and muscle mass, which also benefits your heart and energy levels.

There are many, many other ways to get your body moving and your heart pumping. Consider a few of these options: organized sports such as volleyball or softball, swimming, walking, running, biking, dancing, bowling, golf, yoga, playing with your children, gardening, martial arts, housework of any kind, surfing, tennis, walking stairs, walking to work, volunteer work that requires activity, raking the lawn, kneading bread, washing windows, mowing the lawn, carrying groceries, washing the car, shopping, and even sex. And this is just a partial list. I am sure with some creativity, you could come up with many other things that you could do every day that are active.

It may help to take up things in which the entire family can be involved. Bike-riding is an easy one, but what about hiking, camping, fishing, sledding, snowmobiling, rollerblading, four-wheeling, rock climbing, or skiing? There are also many low-impact activities that, while not necessarily increasing heart rate, certainly increase your activity, such as sewing or quilting, playing an instrument, washing dishes, picking vegetables, or tinkering with home improvements.

One trick is to "believe" that you have energy. Once you convince yourself that you have the energy to take the stairs or walk to the store, and once you actually begin to do these activities on a daily basis, the rest will come naturally. You will start to build stamina and strength. Your energy level will rise. You will start to feel better about yourself and your daily life. Once that all falls into place, you will have established a way of thinking and an approach to life that will benefit your health immensely.

Take the Steps

Let's boil this process down into some simple, easy-to-achieve steps:

1. Take an inventory of your daily life. Keep a journal for a week or so that details your activities. Give yourself credit for chasing the grandkids or carrying groceries. Keep a running total of how much activity (anything that increases your heart rate past your baseline) you undertake every day. We are aiming for 30 to 60 minutes daily of activity that gets your heart rate into the target range. Don't forget to count any time you spend walking to work, climbing stairs, etc.

2. Determine how much activity you need to build into your routine. After you have an idea of where you stand in terms of activity currently, you will have a better idea of how much activity you need to build into your life. For the last few years, the recommendation for exercise was thirty minutes three times a week. Now, researchers believe that this is not enough. They are advocating thirty minutes daily. The change may be due to an error in the initial studies, or it could be due to the fact that we are becoming more and more sedentary in our daily lives in general. Make your daily life as active as possible and then, if you need to, begin a formal exercise regimen.

3. Brainstorm a list of ways to become more active. The list should focus on activities that you would enjoy doing, not just rote exercise that you think you "should" do. Fishing, hiking, biking, gardening, martial arts—it doesn't matter. Anything that gets you moving, elevates your mood, and challenges you. If you are competitive, think about walking or running a marathon. If you are a laid-back homebody, consider gardening or even playing an instrument. If you have a family to consider, take up biking or walking and take everyone along. If you are in a job that requires physical labor, it is quite possible that you are already getting enough activity.

4. Try to incorporate one idea at a time into your daily life. Just because you have a wonderful box of chocolates to choose from, doesn't mean that you need to eat the entire box. Choose one activity to start with and make it a regular part of your routine. When the new level of activity is a well-established part of your daily life, add another. As your energy level and confidence increase, you will find yourself auto-

matically adding more movement. Eventually, you will find the right balance for yourself. Remember that behavioral experts say it takes at least three months for a new habit to become ingrained and natural. Don't give up on a new direction too soon.

5. Enjoy your new-found health and well-being.

Spirituality

Religion, faith, spirituality. These are powerful words with emotional connotations. Everyone has a different interpretation of what these words mean. Every woman has a different emotional attachment to what and how each of these concepts play out in her life. Through the years, women have often played the role of spiritual shaman to their tribe or community. Even when women don't have a formal leadership role with respect to spiritual undertakings, they are the unspoken caretakers of the emotional and spiritual worlds of their children and the children of their society. They are the bearers of consistency and discipline that regulate a child's emotional well-being. They are the sponsors of warmth and love that will nourish the seeds of religion in future generations. Not to say that men can't or don't also play these roles—I don't want to engender reverse bias—but most women excel at them and seek them out.

In our past, women have had a support system to give structure to their lives and social existence. Since the time of the automobile, we have become less dependent on each other as a community, and women are fast losing a dependable structure that serves as a learning institution, as well as an emotional support. Though technology brings us a high standard of living and many creature comforts, it is forcing many changes in our social systems. Without these systems, women have nowhere to turn for advice, support, and nurturing. They have nowhere to practice at developing their own sense of selves. Our young women are increasingly turning to louder and more dangerous rites of initiation and taking difficult paths on the journey to learning about their inner lives.

This is yet another reason to pay special attention to your health, particularly your heart. We have already established that stress is a major factor in developing heart disease. We know that the many addictions we take on in order to soothe our souls are also risky. I believe it is important for everyone, but particularly

One Step at a Time

Researchers have found that exercise done in five-minute increments is just as beneficial as longer periods of exercise. It is also easier to work into your day and for that reason is easier to maintain. Remember that is not just about your heart. It is about your overall health and longevity. You will feel better and everyone around you will feel better knowing that poor health will not take you away from them prematurely. You are worthy of a fulfilling life full of energy and spirit. An active lifestyle will pay untold dividends in the long run, and it starts with just a few stolen moments every day.

women, to take special care to develop their sense of spirituality. Having a strong sense of faith, no matter which religious direction it might take, can serve as a buffer against the daily stresses of life. It can be a stronghold when life becomes difficult. It also serves a very important function that we so often lose sight of, service to others.

If you can summon the energy to take dinner to a sick friend or supply a warm embrace to a conflicted teenager or speak a kind word to a stranger, you will be extending your sense of spirituality in a way that will not "empty" you, but fill you. This sense of filling is at the heart of spirituality. And it serves not only your soul, but the soul of others as well.

There are many theories about the development of spirituality, but there are four clear steps that we all go through. We have the ability to take all of these steps every day in our lives, but they are easily pushed aside in the face of work, family, school, and busy schedules. These four steps have become increasingly apparent in my own life, so I started looking for their place in my patients' lives as well. I was not surprised to see them at work there, as well as at work in the lives of my friends and family. I like to define them in this manner because they are not religion-based. They will fit with whatever form you choose to follow. They are religiously "generic." Follow these steps through with me, and as we go, I think you will see their value and come to understand how they positively impact your heart and your overall health.

Awareness

This is the first step to understanding just about anything in life. If you are not "aware" that you drink too much, you are not likely to stop. If you are not "aware" that you are yelling at your children, you are not likely to seek other ways of communicating. If you are not "aware" that smoking is wreaking havoc on your health, what would be your motivation to stop? Awareness is an integral part of change, as well as growth.

As tiny babies, we all start with about the same level of awareness. We know when we are hungry, tired, or uncomfortable. We soon learn that when we cry, someone comes to alleviate our discomfort. Eventually, we become aware that our helpers are the same one or two people every time. Soon, we are able to identify these people as our parents, and surely the world revolves around us with them in close orbit to tend to our every wish.

As we grow out of infancy and into toddlerhood, we are still at the center of our world, but we start to become aware of a bigger world. It can be at times exciting and scary. It is big and loud and full of things to explore. Our awareness levels expand exponentially at this age.

As we work our way through childhood and into the teen years, we take on a new kind of awareness. We soon learn about ourselves as individuals and test the boundaries of our personality.

As we settle into adulthood, awareness becomes a much more intricate and subtle process. We have assimilated much of our common experiences. Life becomes as much a matter of habit as exploration. We turn our investigations inside. We start to spend more time thinking about matters on a different plane. For some, religion becomes more important. For others, finding a place or sense of belonging becomes paramount. This is where humans get to be completely unique but also totally individual and isolated. Our sense of internal spirit springs from the quest to find a common purpose, but the manner in which we seek it will have as many variations as human nature.

At this point in life, our awareness of our inner nature becomes as important as our awareness of the outer world, and we will have accomplished the first step. This step can actually be accomplished at ANY age, especially in women, but it becomes a matter of "fact" and daily life at this age.

Acceptance

Once we have awareness of inner nature and sense of spirituality, we have to go through the excruciating process of accepting it. Here is an example.

I have a delightful patient that was born into a family that was very religious. They attended church every Sunday and devoted much time, talent, and money to their church. She felt strongly about her faith but related to me that something was always just "off" for her. The family attended a charismatic Christian church. They were very vocal in their worship services, and privacy was not a deeply valued characteristic. This patient happened to be a very private person.

Through her years of growing, she attended her church and loved her family there. However, as she aged and her awareness of her inner spirituality became clearer for her, she started to question the religious direction she was on. She still attended her church faithfully but no longer felt "nurtured" there. The services left her feeling drained and tired. She didn't feel that she was a strong part of the group, because she just wasn't comfortable exposing or sharing herself as easily as others did. She had become aware of an inner characteristic; now she was struggling to accept it.

Eventually, she simply could not make peace with her church's form of worship and explored other options. Eventually, she settled on a more structured service and a church that was "quieter" in its expectations. She told me that from the first moment she stepped into the quiet and somewhat formal atmosphere of the new church, she felt as if she had found something she had been looking for all of her life. By becoming aware of her private nature and accepting it, she was able to put into place a piece of herself that she had always been seeking. She had actually taken the next two steps in her spiritual evolution, acceptance and transformation.

Transformation

This patient's awareness and acceptance led her to take a new direction in life. This step led to what she experienced as a transformation in her life. She was more relaxed and content. She had found a major piece of herself and put it into place.

Many people will have taken the steps of awareness and acceptance. For some, it may be the knowledge that they need to stop drinking. They have accepted that they have a problem. For some people, these steps will come in the form of a quiet longing for something "more" in life, something not materialistic. For many people, transformation will not come until a life-changing event takes place, acting as a catalyst. It may come in the form of "bottoming out," as it would with an addict. It may come in the form of an illness or even a mid-life crisis. Transformation can be the most difficult step. It is where the rubber meets the road and one must actually make the changes. If you are lucky, it will be an easy step. It will come as a relief, as it did for my patient when she changed her church affiliation.

I have seen many patients go through major transformations in their inner nature, particularly when they are faced with a potentially life-threatening illness. For many of them, the illness serves as a catalyst to make changes that they have been aware of and accepted as desirable. They may have been harboring the desire to expand themselves by seeing the world. When they are faced with the possibility of limited time, they transform themselves and their lives to make this possible. I have had patients change jobs or stop working entirely. I have even had a few devote themselves more fully to their careers. Some decide that their families are their top priority, and spending time with them is where they "find themselves." These folks usually rearrange life to place family as a top priority. I have had patients that had no family or strong social connections. They were traditionally loners at heart and were quite satisfied with their solitary life. To my surprise, their transformation took the form of seeking even more solitude. They felt a calling to write a book or compose music. For them, sharing life came in the form of sharing their creativity.

It is difficult to predict the form a transformation will take, but rest assured, it is capable of bringing peace and healing. It becomes a resolution point and provides a new sense of quiet. You can also be assured that it leads to the most important and final step, service.

Service

This is the point where we may agree to disagree. In my philosophy, it is a rock-solid point, but for others it will not be. I could have stopped the discussion at transformation. What does it matter what form the transformation takes as long as it is true and complete? The point of the transformation is to provide reconciliation for the transformed, and that will vary greatly from individual to individual. The outcome of the transformation is not as important as the process.

In a small way I agree with that, but I do think it matters what becomes of the transformation. I think for it to be truly useful and healthy, it must involve an element of service. The greatest sign of spirituality and maturity we can present is that of service. All of the great religions, old and recent, share this common theme. This is the place and time that we step outside of our limited human experience and open up to the greater good. This is where we demonstrate the ability to put our personal selves aside and serve the greater humanity. In doing so, we open ourselves to the world in the largest sense of the word. We transcend ourselves. For me, service is the only form of transcendence that means anything.

There are some who might argue that a hermit who spends his life in the wilderness seeking spiritual truths has accomplished all of the steps of spirituality and come to a greater and bigger world. This may be true, but in what way has that hermit served humanity? What has that person done to improve the world or elevate a soul? Many of the great religious leaders went through periods of contemplation and isolation, but in all cases they "came down off the mountain" in order to serve humanity. Their transformation called them back to the heart of the world so that they might serve a purpose.

And there is the rub. That purpose may be unclear. It may be foggy. It might not be romantic or beautiful. It might be messy and actually quite awful. When I started writing this book, I had a romantic notion of putting my knowledge of medicine down on paper as a way to express my love and concern for my patients and other women struggling with health issues. I envisioned myself as a bit of an artist struggling to express himself in a way that would benefit humanity.

It turns out that writing a book is actually a laborious and somewhat boring process. I still believe that this book serves a purpose beyond myself, but I had to struggle through many months of agonizing writing and editing to produce the finalized pages you now hold in your hand. I don't illustrate this story so that you might give me recognition for my hard work and dedication. I share it so that you might understand that your service may not end up taking the form you think it should.

Let's look at the example of a social worker. A certain young woman started off her education wanting to work in the field of business law. She was intelligent and strong, and most of all, she liked to argue. She felt she was perfectly suited to the practice of law. After a few years in school, she had a niggling in the back of her mind that told her the practice of law just wasn't "enough." She couldn't get close enough to her clients to feel that she was really helping them, and she wasn't really that interested in business after all. She really wanted to help children. She had become aware of a trait that she had not really known of before.

She struggled through two more years of business school and received her diploma. She even started the process of applying to law schools, but her heart wasn't in it. She told herself that she could do volunteer work with kids as a way to help them and still have her career, but eventually she knew that she was just lying to herself. She accepted that her "calling" required her to make kids her career. She decided to seek other options actively. For her, the steps of acceptance, transformation, and service where the same, because she applied for a job as a social worker and was hired by a state agency. After a period of training, she was assigned her own caseload of children and families. Her service to these families became well known. She loved her job and loved the families and served in her position well. She achieved a sense of spirituality through her service at work.

Unfortunately, spirituality is not always so cut and dried. Let's look at an example with respect to health.

I had a patient that was seeing me because one of her heart valves had been destroyed by a diet drug that she had been taking. She was facing a long illness and most likely replacement surgery. I reluctantly shared the news with her and watched the shock and worry settle into her expression. These moments are the most difficult for me, because though I can diagnose and even treat the heart condition, I can do little to soften the impact the news carries. Nor can I do much to help with the emotional healing. I wondered where her spiritual journey would take her.

This was a woman who had struggled with her weight all of her life. She had tried diets, drugs, and even surgery. In the end, it had all caught up with her health. She had come to see herself as her weight. She was so obsessed with her physical image that she had lost sight of her internal image. As is typical, my news was a catalyst for her to do some inner searching.

Through the following months, we worked through her health issues with various drugs and treatments. She had an appointment with me nearly every week for at least four months. It must have been a particularly stressful time for her. One day she came for an appointment. The second I stepped through the door, she broke down in tears. I wasn't sure what was troubling her, so I asked her to tell me what was going on. Why the tears? She explained to me that she realized, after all this time, that food really did nothing for her—it was the struggle and chaos that she latched on to. She was locked in a constant battle with herself. Without it, she felt completely empty.

As we have discussed, feelings of emptiness run deep and are often accompanied by an addiction. I won't dissect her childhood in an attempt to explain the origins of this empty feeling. It is enough to say that she became aware of it and accepted it, possibly for the first time in her life. She had taken the first two steps. I did my best to offer support but knew that the transformation had to come from within her, and I was not surprised to find her in my office in about a month with a story to tell. She had decided to forever rid herself of the struggle. She stopped making menus and diet plans and grocery lists. She went to the store and bought whatever looked good. She didn't worry about what was healthy or "correct" to eat. She simply bought what she wanted, when she wanted it. All of this carried one condition: she could not eat when she felt sad, lonely, or tired. Unfortunately for her, this was the majority of the time. The sadness and loneliness were so familiar to her that she had a difficult time recognizing their pangs when they hit, but with a lot of hard work and some help from a therapist, she was able to do just that. She replaced eating with other "comforting" activities. For her that took the form of reading, writing in her journal, walking her dogs, and vegging out in front of the TV. She had made a transformation.

This story clearly illustrates the first three steps we have talked about, but where is the fourth and final step? The step that I proclaim to be the most important? In this case, it is subtle but so very important. The service was to her family and her children. Because she carved out a piece of health for herself, she was able to offer more to her children. In the past, she would tune them out when she was eating. She just could not be emotionally available for them. Now, though it is still difficult, she makes a conscious effort to pay attention to them on an external and internal level. In the past, she realized that something was missing in her parenting. Her children wanted nothing materialistic, but she felt she was failing to give them what they needed emotionally. How could she show them the best examples of what life should look like when she was engaged in a constant struggle of her own that didn't allow her to support them when they needed it?

Now she realizes that we all struggle, but the struggle takes on a different tone when it is done from a sense of being grounded and an inner sense of self. We are able to struggle and still help others, whether it be through parenting, leading, or loving. In the end, that is all that matters.

CHAPTER 8

The End Is Really a Beginning

Sometimes the Dragon Wins

Because we have been talking about spirituality, I will unveil my struggle and perhaps my greatest weakness. I have yet to accept the fact that sometimes the dragon wins—sometimes my patients die. There is nothing that I, nor modern medicine, can do to help them. They are either too ill or too old and their hearts just won't beat any longer. For me, the most gut-wrenching job I have is to hold the hand of a patient that is dying and to feel their heartbeat slow and fade. It is like watching a piece of myself die. Every time. It is never easy, nor do I expect it ever shall be. I still continue to rail against the injustice of death—the timing, the brutality, the sheer randomness of it. For me, it doesn't matter if my patient is ninety years old and has lived a full life. I still dread the call from her family or the hospital that will tell me she is dying and can I please come?

Watching an elderly patient die with grace and dignity is every bit as difficult as watching a thirty-year-old mother die in the emergency room because, in spite of our best medical efforts, her heart won't start beating again. I wake up every morning wondering if God's finger will reach down that day and take a patient. Will they be young or old? Will I be strong enough to stand by, or will I retreat in panic and shame?

I love the old myths and tales of knights in shining armor and fancy myself to be polished and gleaming from head to toe. I like to walk into an examination room believing, truly believing, that I have the "magic" to heal the ailment about to be presented to me. This piece of fantasy sustains me on days that I am helpless in the face of a greater power. When facing down death, my armor becomes a rusted shell and my skillful medical swordplay becomes a weak attempt at finding a pulse.

I don't know if I will ever accept that death is inevitable. I don't know if I should. I just know that for now, I will not accept it. Maybe even in that, I have found my calling.

A New Beginning

As humans, our struggles become sacred. They are important. They are at the crux of our nature. As humans, we demonstrate ourselves in the way we take on the difficulties presented to us.

As a doctor, I want all of my patients to emerge from their struggles with disease victorious. I want to see them rise from the ashes like a Phoenix. However, I also believe that disease is essential to the human struggle. It is another arena, as undesirable as it may be, that we have an opportunity to face ourselves, fight a battle, and come away with a story to tell.

I cannot be sure the advice contained here will protect your heart entirely. Science and knowledge are still evolving. We are still learning and discovering. In spite of our best efforts, every person is individual and will respond individually. Even if everything I teach works for 99.5% of my patients, there will be a 0.5% that will not be helped. Their hearts have a different story to tell.

If we are fortunate, tomorrow will bring a magic bullet in the form of Teflon armor for the heart. Maybe one small pill will emerge that will protect the heart completely and entirely, forever eradicating heart disease in all of its forms. Until then, we will continue to struggle.

Throughout chapters 3 and 4, we took the time to get to know Sarah, a woman that I hope every reader can relate to. Not necessarily because her life is similar or her battles are similar but simply because she IS fighting, as we all are. She is trying to find a way through life that works for her parents, her husband, her children, and even her coworkers. In all of the ensuing chaos, she forgot about herself. Her heart was forced to find a way to remind her that she was important too. Sarah could have responded in any number of ways, but she chose to slow down, examine life, examine herself, and change her course.

A new beginning.

A New Way

We looked at risk factors and disease processes. We examined ways to make improvements and ways to deal with a negative diagnosis should that day come. For every page on drugs or treatments, we countered with a page on diet and movement. Even in the writing of this book, I searched for balance. I made a concerted effort to practice what I preach, lest the words come through as hollow and meaningless.

In the same way, I hope that you will take these words and make them your own. I hope you will take them into your life and carve a path of change that will bring you to the healthy, fulfilling lifestyle you want for yourself and your family, whatever form that may take. In the beginning, you may follow my advice step by step and avoid veering from the course set out by a "professional." Eventually, you will realize that you are the professional and you will use this book as a foundation to form your own health plan.

A new way.

The Part Can Never Be Well Unless the Whole Is Well

I realize I have spoken frequently about my mother throughout the book. To me it seemed natural. She is the woman that first formed my impression of women. Mostly, she instilled in me a sense of wonder and respect. In spite of my years of medical training, scientific study, and everyday practice, I still feel that everything I know about women I learned from my mother.

As a child, she had many ways of teaching. Some were old-fashioned by today's standards and some were so forward-thinking that she was ahead of her time. Some lessons I took to heart, others I attempted to deflect, but the true genius of her parenting was that she lived and breathed by one simple creed uttered by Plato.

Everything she endeavored to teach me was infused with this truth. Therefore, it didn't matter if I heard or obeyed only a portion of what she said to me. In the end, I still received her teaching in its most distilled form. This truth, I hope, echoes throughout the pages of this book. If your arm is broken, your entire body feels ill. If you are mired in depression, it will reflect in your physical health. Your heart will never be well unless the whole of you is well. This book speaks predominantly about one part of the body, but tending to this one part will, in a greater way, tend to the whole. Thank you for joining me on this journey, and remember…

The part can never be well unless the whole is well.

RESOURCES

Literature Cited

The Seventh Report on the Joint National Committee on Prevention, Detection, Evaluation, and Treatment of High Blood Pressure (JNC 7). 2003. NIH Publication No. 03-5233 (May).

Avas, N. T., D. P. White, J. E. Manson, M. J. Stampfer, F. E. Speizer, A. Malhotra, and F. B. Hu. 2003. A prospective study of sleep duration and coronary heart disease in women. *Arch Intern Med.* (Jan 27) 163(2): 205–9.

Bairey Merz, C. N., B. D. Johnson, B. L. Sharaf, V. Bittner, S. L. Berga, G. D. Braumstein, T. K. Hodgson, K. A. Matthews, C. J. Pepine, S. E. Reis, N. Reichek, W. J. Rogers, G. M. Pohost, S. F. Kelsey, G. Sopko, and WISE Study Group. 2003. Hypoestrogenemia or hypothalmic origin and coronary artery disease in premenopausal women: a report from the NHLBI-sponsored WISE study. *J Am Coll Cardiol.* (Feb 5) 41(3): 413–9.

Beery, T. A. 1995. Gender bias in the diagnosis and treatment of coronary artery disease. *Heart Lung.* (Nov-Dec) 24(6): 427–35.

Chaput, L. A., S. H. Adams, J. A. Simon, R. S. Blumenthal, E. Vittinghoff, F. Lin, E. Loh, K. A. Matthews. 2002. *Am J Epidemiol.* (Dec 15) 156(12): 1092–9.

Karas, R and T. Clarkson. Interpreting the cardiovascular effects of hormone-replacement therapy observed in the WHI: Timing is everything. *Menopausal Medicine.* (Winter) 10(4).

Eisenberg, T., C. Adams, E. C. Riggins, M. Likness. 1999. Smokers' sex and the effects of tobacco cigarettes: Subject-related and physiologic measures. *Nicotin Tob Res.* (Dec) 1(4): 317–24.

Esposito, K, Alessandro Pontillo, Carmen DiPalo, Giovanni Giugliano, Mariangella Masella, Raffaele Marfella, and Dario Giugliano. 2003. Effect

171

of weight loss and lifestyle changes on vascular inflammatory markers in obese women. *JAMA*. 289: 1799–1804.

Grady, D., D. Herrington, V. Bittner et al. 2002. Cardiovascular disease outcomes during 6.8 years of hormone therapy: Heart and Estrogen/Progesetin Replacement Study (HERS II) follow up. *JAMA*. 288: 49–57.

Heart and Stroke Foundation of Canada. 1999. The changing face of heart disease and stroke in Canada 2000.

Shaffer, R. B. and C. Corish. 1998. Cardiac surgery and women. *J Cardiovasc Nurs*. (Jul) 12(4): 14–31.

Hunt, S. C., M. Gwinn, and T. D. Adams. 2003. *Am J of Prev Med*. (Feb) 24(2): 136–42.

Labiche, L. A., W. Chan, and L. B. Morgenstern. 2002. Sex and acute stroke presentation. *Ann Emerg Med*. (Nov) 40(5): 453–60.

Levy, D., S. Kenchaiah, M. G. Larson, E. J. Benjamin, M. J. Kupka, K. K. Ho, J. M. Murabito, R. S. Vasan. 2003. Long-term trends in the incidence of and survival with heart failure. *New Engl J Med*. 347:1397–1402.

Lloyd, G. W., N. R. Patel, E. McGing, A. F. Cooper, D. Brennand-Roper, G. Jackson. 2000. Does angina vary with the menstrual cycle in women with premenopausal coronary artery disease? *Heart*. (Aug) 84(2): 189–92.

Longo, L. D. 1997. An imperative in women's health research. Who will pay? *Women's Health Issues*. (Nov-Dec) 7(6):407–9.

Maruccio, E., N. Loving, S. K. Bennett, S. N. Hayes. 2003. A survey of attitudes and experiences of women with heart disease. *Women's Health Issues*. (Jan-Feb) 13(1): 23–31.

McDermott, M. M., P. Greenland, K. Liu, M. H. Criqui, J. M. Guralnik, L. Celic, C. Chan. 2003. Sex differences in peripheral arterial disease: leg symptoms and physical functioning. *J Am Geriatr Soc*. (Feb) 51(2): 222–8.

Nelson, H. D., L. L. Humphrey, P. Nygren, S. M. Teutsch, and J. D. Allan. 2002. Postmenopausal hormone-replacement therapy: scientific review. *JAMA*. (Aug 21) 288(7): 872–81.

Ridker, P. M., J. E. Buring, N. R. Cook, N. Rifai. 2003. C-reactive protein, the metabolic syndrome, and risk of incident cardiovascular events: an 8-year follow-up of 14,719 initially healthy American women. *Circulation*. (Jan 28) 107(3): 391–7.

Schmitz, K. H., D. R. Jacobs, P. J. Schreiner, et. al. The impact of becoming a parent on physical activity: the CARDIA Study. Presented at the American Heart Association's 39th Annual Conference on Cardiovascular Disease Epidemiology and Prevention. March 24-27. Orlando, Fl.

Sdringola, S., D. Patel, and K. L. Gould. 2001. High prevalence of myocardial perfusion abnormalities on positron emission tomography in asymptomatic persons with a parents or sibling with coronary artery disease. *Circulation*. (Jan 30) 103(4): 496–501.

Shumaker, C. Legault, S. R. Rapp, L. Thal, R. B. Wallace, J. K. Ockene, S. L. Hendrix, B. N. Jones, A. R. Assaf, R. D. Jackson, J. M. Kotchen, S. Wassertheil-Smoller, J. Wactawski-Wende, WHMS Investigators. 2003. Estrogen plus progestin and the incidence of dementia and mild cognitive impairment in postmenopausal women: the Women's Health Initiative Memory Study: a randomized controlled trial. *JAMA*. (May 28) 289(20): 2651–62.

Storch, K. F. 2002. Extensive and divergent circadian gene expression in liver and heart. Nature, advanced online publication, doi:10.1038/*Nature* 744 (2002). Waley, Dana et al. 2002. Presentation to the Radiological Society of North America December 4, 2002.

Vittinghoff E, MG Shlipak, PD Varosy, CD Furberg, CC Ireland, SS Khan, R Blumenthal, E Barrett-Connor, S Hulley 2003. Risk factors and secondary prevention in women with heart disease: The Heart and Estrogran/progestin Replacement Study. *Annals of Internal Medicine*. (Jan21) 138(2): 150-1.

Vongpatanasin, W., M. Tuncel, Z. Wang, D. Arbique, B. Mehrad, I. Jialal. 2003. Differential effects of oral versus transdermal estrogen replacement therapy on C-reactive protein in postmenopausal women. *J Am Coll Cardiol*. (Apr 16) 41(8): 1358–63.

Weintraub, W. S. and V. Vaccarino. 2003. Explaining racial disparities in coronary outcomes in women. *Circulation*. (Sep 2) 108(9): 1041–3.

Smoking Cessation Resources

Here are some web links to some great sites with further information about smoking cessation.

National Center for Disease Control: Comprehensive information on smoking and tobacco. Lots of help for those looking to quit smoking.
http://www.cdc.gov/tobacco/

American Lung Association: Their Freedom from Smoking campaign has been very successful. Lots of helpful information here.
http://www.lungusa.org/tobacco/smkcessafac99.html

QuitNet: This website sponsors an online community of those looking to quit smoking. Get support from others on their discussion boards.
http://www.quitnet.com/

SmokeFree: This website is sponsored by five different government agencies. It is a very informative site offering a wide range of services.
http://smokefree.gov/

Women's Heart Health Sites

Heart Center Online: http://www.heartcenteronline.com

American Heart Association: http://women.americanheart.org

National Institute of Health: http://hin.nhlbi.nih.gov/womencvd/

www.womenheart.org

www.hadassah.org

www.blackwomenshealth.org

www.hispanichealth.org

www.healthywomen.org

www.ywca.org

INDEX OF COMMON TESTS

Blood tests: Blood drawn from a vein. Can test for cholesterol levels, cardiac enzymes, oxygen level, Prothrombin Time and International Normalize Ratio, as well as other markers for heart disease.

Electrocardiography (EKG): Noninvasive, painless test that measures heart rate and waves. May come in the from an exercise stress test as well.

Chest X-Ray: Used to examine heart and lungs. Determines size and shape of the heart, presence of calcium deposits, and lung condition.

Nuclear Scanning: Radioactive dyes are injected into the veins and measured. Demonstrates heart chamber size, tracks blood flow, and measures pumping ability of the ventricles. Subtests include radionuclide ventriculogram and exercise perfusion scan.

Echocardiography: A sonogram-like test that looks at the heart's pumping strength as well as heart size, valve problems, blood flow patterns, and heart structure.

Catheterization and Angiography: Invasive procedure using catheters to visually examine the heart, ventricles, and vessels.

Electrophysiology: Invasive test where a catheter is threaded into the heart' chamber. Measures the electrical activity of the heart.

CT, MRI, and PET Scans: Noninvasive scanning techniques that produce "pictures" of the heart and surrounding structures.

Commonly-Prescribed Cardiac Drugs

Nitrates: These drugs are used primarily to treat angina pain and occasionally to manage a heart attack. Most widely used drug is nitroglycerin. Some brand names are Nitro-Bid, Isordil, and Nitrogard.

Beta-Blockers: Also used for angina pain but also blood pressure. Some brand names are Lopressor, Tenormin, Betapace.

Calcium Channel Blockers: Used for angina pain and to lower blood pressure. Commonly used brands are Norvasc, Procardia, and Cardizem.

Thrombolytics: These drugs dissolve clots and restore blood flow through obstructed vessels. Brand names include Activase, Retavase, and Streptase.

Lipid-Lowering: These drugs lower cholesterol levels by holding bile acids in the intestine, inhibiting them from entering the bloodstream. Common names are Colestid, Lopid, Mevacor, Pravachol, Zocor, Lipitor, and Lescol.

Anti-Hypertensives: These medications lower blood pressure. Brand names might include Aldomet, Catapres, and Hytrin.

ACE Inhibitors: Used to manage heart failure. Names include Capoten, Zestril, Prinivil, Accupril, Lotensin, Monopril, Altace, and Mavik.

Diuretics: Also used to manage heart failure by removing excess water from the body. Brand names include Zaroxolyn, Aldactone, and Diuril. Spironolactone, Triamterene, and Amiloride are examples of combination medications that also manage potassium levels.

Inotropic Agents: Digitalis and digoxin increase the heart's squeezing ability, which determines the amount of blood it can pump.

Antiarrhythmic Agents: Correct rhythm abnormalities. Common names are Xylocaine, Norpace, Cardioquin, and Adenocard.

Anticoagulants: Reduce the blood's ability to clot. Commonly prescribed are Coumadin, Lovenox, and Fragmin.

INDEX

0-595-29743-9